The Opioid Epidemic Consumers & HealthCare Guide

VIII

PREPUBLICATION COMMENTS AND REVIEWS FOR
THE OPIOID EPIDEMIC CONSUMERS & HEALTHCARE GUIDE

The book is exceptionally comprehensive, addressing issues of importance to both professionals and the public. It is divided into discrete chapters that address important issues related to the management of pain and the opioid crisis. Each chapter includes appropriate references that can also serve as sources of additional information. The book includes a significant number of useful appendices.

- **John L. Melvin, M.D.**, **MMSc.** Emeritus Professor and Chair, Department of Rehabilitation Medicine, Sidney Kimmel Medical College at Thomas Jefferson University. Past president of American Academy of PM&R.

I have read Dr. Foster's book and found it to be excellent. It is both factual with clear data but also personal and practical. I think he presents a very balanced review of the topic that has become very political, emotional, and one-sided. Congratulations on this excellent book!

- **Prof. Gerard A. Malanga, M.D.** Rutgers School of Medicine, NJ Medical School. Author of four textbooks - Last one 2017: **"Regenerative Treatments in Sports and Orthopedic Medicine."** Incoming president of the Interventional Orthopedic Foundation (IOF) in 2019.

This book is a clearly written, comprehensive examination of an important problem. Written by an experienced clinician, the book is thorough and thoughtful. Each chapter is sprinkled with charts and facts yet written in clear, non- technical language that is very readable even with no medical background. For the health care professional there is a very useful listing of "References, Recommended Readings and Resources" at the end of each chapter. This book should become a core textbook in every Pain Fellowship. In fact, in view of the widespread reality of our opioid epidemic, I would recommend this book to every medical student and practicing physician.

- **Jacqueline Wertsch, M.D.,** Professor Emeritus of Physical Medicine and Rehabilitation. Medical College of Wisconsin. Milwaukee, Wisconsin.

I am very impressed. It is well-written and well researched. Thank you for allowing me to review this book. This information is very much needed in the public sphere. I hope you gain a wide readership!

- **Daniel McDevitt, M.D.,** Peachtree Vascular Specialists, Stockbridge GA. Asst. Clinical Professor, Dept. of Surgery Medical College of GA, Atlanta Medical Center and Emory University Hospital Midtown.

Dr. Foster has undertaken the monumental task of helping the layman and healthcare professional to understand the opioid epidemic. He succeeds in laying out a systematic analysis of the scope of this multifactorial problem.

Dr. Foster incorporates recent data, historical perspectives and commonly held misconceptions about the causes of the opioid crisis. He effectively exposes the truth, and in the process lays the groundwork for future actions to prevent recurrences. This book is an excellent source of information and education written by a Pain Management physician who lives on the front line of the opioid epidemic.

- **Carlos J. Giron M.D.** Founder and past president of The Georgia Society of Interventional Pain Physicians (GSIPP). Founder and CEO of the Pain Institute of Georgia, and Macon Pain Center.

I found this to be a well-researched, well-written, balanced, data driven comprehensive look at the opioid epidemic. Although I was familiar with many aspects of this problem, I also learned a lot reading through the manuscript. I like the fact that you do not sugar coat the problem, explode a few myths with the use of statistics, and also make it clear that we "can't throw out the baby with the bath water" and that while we have to seek and implement solutions, there is still a need for prescribing to certain patients. I certainly see the value of the book for healthcare providers as well as the general public and commend you on this accomplishment.

- **Dr. Clover Hall, Ed.D.** Educator (Retired).

This book is informative and relatively easy to read. One of the things I liked most about the book is that although it relies heavily on research and data collected on the subject of opioid treatment and abuse, it does not overwhelm the reader with scientific terms and expressions.

Overall, the book is a valuable tool in the war against the opioid epidemic and if it gets in the hands of enough people who work in the field or have loved ones whose lives have been derailed by the crisis, it should help to save some lives.

- **Howard Jackson Jr**. Senior Manager, Information and Communications Technology

---

A must read, and not just for professionals, but for everyone!!

Dr. Foster gives an interesting and provocative account of the dynamics of the opioid epidemic on our society. The book is relatable to any reader since the opioid epidemic has touched, or will touch just about everyone, whether family member, friend, co- worker, patient, client. I found it applicable to my area of practice of child welfare law, and my personal observation on the effect on the elderly as it relates to pain management.

- **Hazel Langrin-Robertson, Esq**

I am truly impressed by the thoroughness and details presented. Your first-hand knowledge and experience as a Pain Management Doctor, blended with your compassion for people, your solution and result oriented thinking make this a must read book. To me, it offers perspective relevant to those who legislate as well as offer an opportunity to inform and create awareness and solution amongst socially conscious members of our society.

- **Andrea Owen-Boyd:** Financial consultant.

As a mid-level provider practicing in the field of pain management, the detailed information and data Dr. Foster provides regarding the current opioid epidemic we're facing is both eye-opening and insightful. All of the given data is not only credible, but will henceforth alter my approach to managing pain. Congratulations on such a wonderful accomplishment.

- **Chantel Lee**, Physician Assistant.

The author's intent to bring awareness to consumers was definitely executed if read by consumers, family, friends and healthcare professionals.

I strongly believe this book will be beneficial to the other desired target audience "healthcare professionals." Bringing this epidemic out in the limelight will definitely help these professionals better assist those affected directly or indirectly. Again, awareness is essential for explaining to professionals how to deal with this epidemic. Overall, I found this book very informative and it has opened my eyes to the use of opioids which is often prescribed to myself for my military injuries that are now causing chronic pain.

- **Michael Thompson, Lieutenant Colonel (Retired), US Army**

This book is an easy read for anyone who has an interest in acute or chronic pain. This includes health care providers who may be just curious to those who are pain specialist. Those who are directly or indirectly affected by opioids will find comfort in knowing that you are not alone. This book allows the reader to have an excelled understanding of the epidemic and more importantly, resources to get help for those in need.

- **Santhosh Thomas, DO, MBA,** Associate Medical Director, Richard E. Jacobs (REJ) Health Center; Medical Director, Center for Spine Health – REJ; Co-Director Medical Spine Fellowship. Cleveland Clinic, Avon, Ohio.

I have just reached Chapter 15 of the book. I can tell you today, that even if I don't get to read another page of it, I have found this book to be brilliantly conceived, thoroughly researched and ingeniously presented. It paints a very vivid picture of what I know to be factual. It addresses a very important issue that we face today. It answers questions that we may have now or could have in the future. Thank you for inviting me to be a part of it!

- **Janie B. Pope, RN**

This is an insightful educational guide to helping the addict, caregiver and/or healthcare provider better understand and defeat the opioid crisis. As a healthcare provider, I have witnessed first-hand the devastation this crisis has caused in families. It is a privilege and our responsibility to pass this wonderful information on to others who may never pick up a book of any kind to read. I highly recommend this book to persons from all walks of life in an effort to combat the opioid crisis facing our communities, state and world. Our communities throughout the world will be a better place because of such a challenging book dedicated to reaching one person at a time saving or changing lives.

- **Dottie Borders, MSW, CM**, Medical Social Worker.

In this masterful work, Dr. Foster takes us on a comprehensive analysis of the American opioid crisis. It is well organized, presented by the history of the crisis with the involvement of the pharmaceutical industry, the doctors, policies and other healthcare providers, all having an impact on the current opioid epidemic. It is very informative. It is a great resource for practicing providers. Strongly recommend this book for all providers involved in pain management.

- **Angella Green, FNP,** Keizer Family Medicine, Salem, Oregon.

My overall impression is that this is a well-researched, balanced and broadly applicable treatment of the subject matter. I am particularly impressed by its conversational tone and clear appeal to the entire spectrum of stakeholders. It is a work whose time has well and truly come and I feel confident that it will do well. Impressive work Dr. Foster.

- **Dr. Brian James, BSc, MBBS, DA, FRCA** Anaesthetist, Bustamante Hospital for Children, Bustamante Hospital Operating Theatre Users Committee Chairman. Kingston, Jamaica W.I.

TO ALL THE REVIEWERS

THANK YOU ALL SO MUCH FOR CONTRIBUTING YOUR TIME AND EFFORT IN REVIEWING THIS BOOK INDEPENDENTLY BEFORE ITS PUBLICATION.

YOU HAVE MADE THIS BOOK SO MUCH BETTER THAN I COULD HAVE BY MYSELF.

I AM TRULY GRATEFUL TO EACH AND EVERYONE OF YOU............... DTF.

The Opioid Epidemic Consumers & HealthCare Guide

D. TERRENCE FOSTER, M.D., FAAPMR, DABPM

Global Health and Consortium Publishing.

GHC^P

Copyright © 2018 by D Terrence Foster, MD

Publisher: Global Health and Consortium . PO Box 824, Morrow, GA 30260.

GHCpublishing.com

GHC^P

Printed in the United States of America. No claim to Original United States Government Work.

First published in January 2019.

Library of Congress Cataloging in Publication Data

The Opioid Epidemic Consumers & HealthCare Guide
D Terrence Foster. M.D

1SBN:13 978-1-7328804-0-5 (Paperback).

Library of Congress Control Number: 2018912167

Also available:
1SBN:13 978-1-7328804-1-2 (eBook)
 1SBN:13 978-1-7328804-2-9 (Hardback)

X

Acknowledgments

The writing of this book is a total collaboration of many different forces coming together. I want to take the opportunity to thank my beloved wife Maxine, who shared in the sacrifice of this project coming to completion.

To my present staff (CPARM and Personal Injury Solutions), particularly our practice administrator, Mrs. Arlene Soriano and my PA, Jennifer Garrett. I have learned a lot from you all and continued to learn. You have helped to provide clarity even when I am at my best.

If I sometimes seem unmoved, unshakable and display a sense of calmness even in what may be considered as chaotic, it is because of the many great teachers I have had both as a student and as a professional. Over the years I have also learned from my former students, colleagues, but most of all from countless patients that I have allowed to teach me. The medical profession is a never-ending and growing Web of knowledge; I am so grateful for the power of learning and so many who have contributed to my growth.

Special thanks also to everyone who participated in our free/uncompensated, honest, independent and impartial prepublication review of this book. I am truly appreciative for the time that you have contributed as well your excellent constructive comments and reviews that you have provided. You have made this book significantly better than I could by myself alone. Those of you who were unable to participate I do understand and appreciate you as well. Any criticism of this book rests solely on my shoulders and no one else.

A significant number of references are from the governmental press or publication releases, research or data collections. I find it necessary to give special thanks to the many great scientists, researchers, and assistants who work in government agencies. Without their work, many of the things that we do today would not be possible. I am truly grateful.

There are no commercial or sponsoring entity or relevant conflicting disclosure associated with this book.

XII

Disclaimer

This publication is intended to inform and educate consumers and medical providers in general. The subject matter encompasses many areas related to the opioid epidemic as well as specific disciplines associated or incorporated in the subject matter. Also, the subject matter continues to change and evolve. Because of these reasons and others, readers are advised to consult with their own personnel for medical and/or legal advice where appropriate.

Also, this book covers many states; the laws of each state are different, and may not necessarily reflect the readers' state of residence. The author has taken great care in researching and presenting the facts in this book. Every effort has been made to ensure that this book is free of error. Regardless, the author and publisher do not assume any responsibilities or liabilities for errors or omission. Also, all liabilities are disclaimed from using any or part of the information from this book.

The use of brand names as opposed to generic names sometimes appear in this book (for example Xanax, Valium, Tylenol, Soma, and others) often because of greater familiarity to the public/consumers rather than any specific associated or related negative factors pertaining to the pharmaceutical companies or manufacturers of these drugs or products.

For the numerous references, recommended reading and resources that are listed, every effort has been made to obtain and give credit for all the material that we have used that required copyright release, and even those that did not. If for any reason, any content that appears in this book that does not have the author's or publishers' permission, we apologize for the error of omission and ask that you contact us for corrective action.

Dedication

To my mom, who has shown more strength than anyone should have.

To Nia: whom I will always love. I know that you will turn your life around. I have allowed you to teach me that I should "never try to gain the love of anyone by giving up loving yourself." I truly hope you have learned the same, too.

Table of Contents

Introduction

The Opioid Epidemic

The opioid epidemic or crisis is one of the most significant epidemics in the modern era. The Centers for Disease Control and Prevention (CDC) stated that more than 632,000 people have died from drug overdoses between 1999 and 2016.

In most of these deaths, 66% involved opioids. About 40% of all opioid deaths involved prescription opioids such as OxyContin or oxycodone HCl, hydrocodone, and morphine. Non-prescription opioids such as illegal heroin and illicitly manufactured fentanyl (IMF) accounted for most of the deaths, or about 60%. More than 63,000 people died in 2016 alone from drug overdoses; and of this number, more than 42,000 died from opioids. These included prescription opioids, heroin, IMF and its analogs which resulted in a total number of deaths five times higher than in 1999.

The economic burden and healthcare costs continue to rise. The National Academy of Medicine (NAM) formally called the Institute of Medicine estimates that over 100 million Americans are suffering from chronic pain, costing the economy upwards of $635 billion per year. The Council of Economic Advisers or National Economic Council estimated that in the year 2015, the costs to the economy for the opioid epidemic, related deaths and overdoses was $504 billion.

The use of opioids for the treatment of chronic pain has been at the center of the controversy related to the epidemic. Many have attributed the rising number of deaths to escalating opioid prescriptions, which date back to the late 1990s.

Between 1999 and 2010, prescription-drug sales to doctors, healthcare providers, pharmacies and healthcare facilities quadrupled, according to the CDC. With that came a parallel increase in opioid overdoses, related deaths, addictions, economic and social burdens.

Prescription opioids peaked in 2010. It continues to decline by about 18% by the end of 2015 although it still remains high relative to 1999 numbers.

Despite the decreasing number of deaths from prescribed opioids, overdose numbers continue to increase, without any clear end in sight. It is now projected that the total deaths from opioid overdose in 2017 will exceed 49,000, while total overdose deaths from all drugs related will exceed 72,000.

Who Should Read this Book and Why?

This book attempts to provide a simple approach and understanding for consumers, the public as a whole, and healthcare providers regarding some of the challenges involved with opioid use and addiction. It will look at the opioid epidemic in general; and treatment options that will be useful in helping those who may be affected or, at some point, be involved in or have relatives/friends or associates who may be victims of this epidemic. It also looks at prevention and some of the obstacles faced by those of us who work with patients who are in pain and/or addicted to some of these medications.

This book's initial development and its draft were primarily meant for general consumers. A deliberate effort was made to avoid some jargon or concepts that may be challenging for them. But as the project developed, it became necessary to produce a book that can and will have significant benefits for healthcare providers as well.

This book is not intended for scholars or those who consider themselves experts or authorities on pain management or addiction medicine. I myself am an expert or authority on these subjects, but of course, I realize I'm not the only one. I fully believe that most of the information provided in this book will be useful to a broad cross-section of the general public. I do understand the limitations of this book and, most significantly, the importance of the subject matter and the depth and breadth to which it extends.

Anyone of the subject title or subtitles that I have discussed can be a title and/or titles of many books and publications. Despite these limitations, I have decided that the best title should be:

The Opioid Epidemic Consumers & HealthCare Guide

This book covers a wide range of topics and issues related to the opioid epidemic, some of which are fairly basic, while others are complex. The content of this book is based primarily on real-life situations, challenges, and outcomes in managing patients who are treated with opioids and other controlled substances, as well as those that are addicted to opioids.

The perspective given in part is from those of us who spend our lives working and caring for them. This book is not a summary obtained by the author from interviewing individuals who work in the field of pain management or addiction medicine or from those who may have a cursory knowledge about the practice of the discipline of pain management and addiction medicine. This is a compressive approach to the opioid epidemic that looks at many angles based on real experiences.

As I've indicated, the need for consumer awareness was a driving force in writing this book. As such, some topics are covered with them in mind. However, although it is not surprising, there is a significant gap between the basic knowledge and understanding of some healthcare providers concerning pain management and treating so-called pain patients. More than 50% of all opioids and controlled substances are prescribed by these providers, which consist of family practice and internal medicine physicians' providers, and their mid-level providers – physician assistants, nurse practitioners, and clinical nurse specialists. They are at the front lines of treating these patients across the country, sometimes in underserved areas. Hence, they are extremely vital in providing medical care in places where healthcare access is limited and very few providers are available to serve these areas.

I believe that the information in this book, although simplified to some degree, will be of benefit to some of them as well as others. By "others," I have included anyone involved in a healthcare capacity or related service, such as medical doctors/ providers, physician assistants, nurse practitioners, nurses, counselors, therapists, aides to these professionals, community leaders, coaches, providers of addiction-medicine support and treatment services, and finally, parents and family members who care. This book is intended for virtually everyone, and that shouldn't surprise many of us; we have an epidemic with such an extremely high probability, that it could potentially affect everyone, and lead to devastating consequences.

This book may never reach the hands of potential substance abusers or those who are likely to become addicts, or who are already addicts. However, if it reaches those of you who are looking out for them and must deal with the challenges of drug addiction and are trying to find ways to improve the lives of others, in the end, our contribution to changing the course of this opioid epidemic can make a difference.

I strongly recommend those who use the information contained here to expand on their knowledge by reading some of the references, recommended reading and resources provided in this book, which will start the process for you.

Don't Get Stuck on a Few Words or
Be Afraid of Reading this Book!

I know that we are all at different levels in life in terms of educational attainment, social status, and professional achievement. But I also know that some of the smartest people in the world have never spent a single day in college; and if they were given the opportunities to master some of the things that those considered "smart" or "learned," they may have done equally well or much better in many instances.

So, if you are a consumer seeking to educate yourself about the opioid epidemic and you look at this book, do not be dismayed by the graphs, tables, numbers, and sometimes maybe words or phrases that you can't pronounce or may not understand. It may seem challenging. However, I urge you not to let that stop you from exploring what I believe and know that you're capable of doing. *In fact, from some of the pre-publication reviews completed it was said that this book is educational and fun to read particularly after the first few chapters.* Every graph and every table come with an explanation. In some instances, even if you do not fully understand the descriptions of graphs or charts, there will be some great basic and useful information that are discussed and presented throughout this book.

I guarantee you will broaden your understanding and knowledge. This will enable you to address better the issues relating to the people you care about. Every effort has been made for the readers of this book to understand the essential idea and information about the opioid epidemic.

If you are a healthcare provider or someone who works in a related capacity, this book should be an easy read, and hopefully, add to your knowledge base and understanding of some of the subtle but important aspects of the fight against the opioid epidemic. On this matter of totally getting the ideas and understanding the information contained in this book, I leave you with the following thought as we all have to challenge ourselves regardless of our endeavors in our daily lives:

The capacity that we have to do anything, whether we believe in our ability or that of others, is often determined by how committed we are in challenging our own beliefs.

Why is This Book Important?

In today's world, we are bombarded with ever-increasing sources of information. The challenge for just about everyone is how quickly and accurately we access and process the information contained in these sources. Our attention span is limited to the extent of what we think is important to us. Even then, we just "don't have time for that."

If any of us were to take the time to access and process the many excellent resources available on the subject matter, this book would be, in part, irrelevant. However, the time needed for anyone to do that would be significant, even for the most learned and sophisticated among us. This means government sources and others — for example, the CDC, National Institutes of Health (NIH), Food and Drug Administration (FDA), Drug Enforcement Administration (DEA), Department of Health and Human Services (HHS), Substance Abuse and Mental Health Services Administration (SAMHSA), National Center on Addiction and Substance Abuse , and the National Institute on Drug Abuse (NIDA), to name a few — are rarely fully utilized by professionals, let alone the general public. In fact, it is a good chance that most consumers would not be familiar with any of these or be familiar with very few of these agencies or associations. Odds are some of them would be more familiar with the "Molly Percocet" song. It would not surprise me if, for example, most physicians and healthcare providers rarely visit their State Medical Board or their malpractice insurance websites, although those also may be excellent sources of information.

Therefore, the vast majority of the public is unlikely to benefit directly from the wealth of available information, even with much effort on the part of various organizations/associations to educate the public or consumers on our country's opioid epidemic.

Hence, the challenge to all of us is that we have to be our brother's keeper. We must be the ones who pay attention to the people we love and care about, primarily because most of them probably won't know or understand when they need help. This book may never get in the hands of a current or future drug addict, but we can be part of the solution for someone in need. This book may be an asset at the time of their most significant need.

I hope that this will provide some meaningful information that will be the gateway to a better understanding of the epidemic or, at the very least, get some people to take vital action in dealing with it. If nothing else, let the discussion begin about some of the issues related to the opioid epidemic that people seldom speak about.

Using Data and Statistics

The understanding of the opioid epidemic in part relies to a significant degree on data collection, statistics, and the conclusions we draw from them. It is important to realize that precise data and, at times, its collection has many factors that influence it. Of course, these will impact the conclusion we can make from the available statistics. It is therefore necessary to analyze and interpret these numbers in gross terms rather than precise concepts or ideas. Imagine statistics such as the total number of opioid-related deaths (both prescribed and illicitly manufactured or illegal drugs) in the United States in 2016, which was 42,249. This number would have been obtained from numerous municipalities, medical examiners and/or other departments responsible for keeping statistics of these deaths throughout the United States. So, what are the odds of these numbers being accurate?

Sometimes, it is also difficult for medical examiners or pathologists to determine which substance is most likely responsible for drug overdoses. There are many reasons, such as multiple drugs being present in the body, various comorbidities, and inconclusive data/laboratory results (among others), contributing to the difficulty in determining a definitive cause of death.

The nature of data collection and processing is lengthy particularly in these cases, and very often we are looking at data from incidents that have occurred several months prior, or sometimes well over a year. We then take the information from those past incidents and make predictions and decisions now that we hope will be reasonable and probably correct.

The point I am making is that a broader perspective is more important than precise numbers that inherently have a very low probability of being accurate.

Other factors often have to be considered: data must be collected, then entered and computed correctly, which allows for other errors. When we look at some data, we often look at them in time frames or data points.

For example, one may look at the number of people who died between July 1, 2016, and June 30, 2017, and would report the number of deaths within that time frame. One may also report on a different point in time between 2016 and 2017, for example, October 1, 2016, and September 30, 2017, and get a different result. All of these may be referred to as 2016 data although they're collected at different points in time. This can be confusing even if they are technically correct and with the appropriate date stated. Unless of course, you are following the methodology very closely.

Having said all of that, most of the collected and used data regarding this epidemic is by government agencies. This process is very tedious and laborious, requiring many hours of processing and utilizing data in ways that are rational. That can sometimes create another set of problems depending on the scientists/researchers' biases, goals or objectives. Therefore, the scientists/researchers' plans are critical in part because many reasonable and different conclusions can often be drawn and also be supported by the same available data.

Because of the nature of the nature of data collection and analysis and the high level at which this has to be done, regardless of our criticism or idealism, we have to use and rely on the data we have as it is simply our best option.

Familiarize Yourself with the Appendices

I have included appendices to facilitate a better understanding and a more enjoyable reading of this book. It is advised that you familiarize yourself with each appendix before reading the main texts of the book.

Although looking at each appendix and knowing what is there, is not a prerequisite to understanding most of the concepts. It will, however, add clarity to some of the information that some of you may encounter for the first time.

The appendices include: How to Calculate Morphine Milligrams Equivalent (MME) Per Day, A Summary of CDC Guidelines for Chronic Opioid Use – 2016, Drugs Schedule **(I – V)** by the DEA, Foster's Opioid Classification Addiction Status or FOCAS, Tables and Charts of frequently used and abused opioids, controlled substances, illegal drugs, and other drugs.

Using the References, Recommended Readings, and Resources

In writing this book, I tried to stay somewhere between providing useful information for consumers and doing the same for healthcare providers. That task wasn't necessarily the easiest thing to accomplish; in some aspect, the material gets a little too complicated for consumers, and it may get too simple (and therefore less useful) for healthcare providers, falling short of what is considered a scholarly book. So, what I've done concerning the **References, Recommended Readings and Resource**s is to use references where they are most likely to be helpful to those wishing to expand their knowledge base, obtain another perspective, or corroborate what I have presented.

I've also included **Recommended Readings and Resources** from the internet that were generated by print, television, and cable media. Sometimes, they take the form of a video or part of a documentary.

I believe that it is more likely that consumers will relate to some of the media-related source articles, resources, and references as opposed to from scientific journals. I do believe that there are very few consumers in general who would be interested in or spend any of their time reading scientific journals. In fact, when I was a resident physician, I can remember we all had to attend required "Journal Club" to encourage and facilitate learning from scientific journals. I doubt much has changed since.

I have spent a significant amount of time reviewing, cross-referencing and reading some of these articles in-depth. However, there are some that I have not read thoroughly or materials and references in articles that I haven't cross-referenced.

I still believe that the ones that are presented here will give additional insight into some of the covered topics. Using these articles from the media can sometimes be challenging if you have little to no background knowledge or foundational information that allows you to process what's being presented. Some of these articles are well-written, while others fall short. Sometimes it appears that the primary objective is to create attention-grabbing headline rather than to present the substance of the article/topic itself. These topics are extremely wide and varied; no single article or even a book can cover any of these topics to the depth that would be considered complete. I've also included a section at the back of the book, referred to as **Useful Resources and Websites**, that will be helpful in understanding the opioid epidemic and becoming a part of the fight against this epidemic, rather than being a victim of its course and impact.

What Makes Me Think I Can Write a Book Like This?

Finally, I decided to write this book because of the knowledge that I've acquired in the field of healthcare, particularly medicine, after practicing as a medical doctor for more than 20 years. Specifically, I am Board Certified in Physical Medicine and Rehabilitation as well as Board Certified in Pain Medicine. I am still practicing, and I am the Chief Medical Officer of a licensed pain clinic where addiction medicine and treating patients with addiction is also part of our practice. I previously served as the Medical Director of an Acute Inpatient Rehabilitation Center for ten years. That Center had a considerable number of patients who were suffering with or had significant acute pain as well as chronic pain. In addition, I have also worked in skilled nursing facilities for several years, caring for the elderly.

I must say that I have been truly fortunate to have passed through some of the most excellent institutions of learning that any physician can ask for in a lifetime. For full disclosure, it is essential to let you know that this book is not a reflection or a description of how I practice medicine in our office and in our state; or relates to anyone I know, specifically in the fields of pain management or addiction medicine.

Also, many have written or become experts on a subject matter after having had direct experience with that subject. With respect to me, I was asked to try a cigarette when I was around 13 or 14 years old. I took a couple of puffs, or so I thought. But for about five minutes after that, I had a significant coughing spell. Since then, I have not smoked another cigarette. I have never tried or used marijuana, although I have had many friends who would smoke it while I was in their company. I don't really have an explanation as to why I didn't; it was not because my parents had some strong denunciation about marijuana or any drugs. It just didn't happen. I was never exposed to illicit drugs such as cocaine, methamphetamine, heroin, phencyclidine or PCP, and others. Neither did I know of anyone or had any friends who traded or used those drugs. My street cred may be limited with respect to direct use, but my professional experience involves interacting with and treating many in the population that I'm now writing about.

It is my intention that this book will make a difference in some people's lives, or in the lives of those we hold close and are most dear to us. If through this book, I can help to save the life of one person, keep one family together, or prevent one baby from being addicted to opioids before taking the first breath of life, I would have accomplished something worthwhile.

Part One

FROM THE START OF THE OPIOID EPIDEMIC TO WHERE WE ARE NOW

Chapter 1

What is This Opioid Epidemic About, and How Did It Start?

The scientific evidence and statistics that exist today clearly support the conclusion that we are in one of the most significant epidemics of our generation, if not the most significant. It is called the opioid epidemic, or narcotic epidemic ('opioid' is also called 'narcotic'). This epidemic has created one of the most devastating health crises in the modern era.[1,10]

We are not alone in fighting an opioid epidemic or crisis. Canada and the USA account for the world's largest percentage of opioid usage in the world.[37] In 2017, it was estimated that approximately 4,000 people in Canada died from an opioid overdose. About 72% of those deaths were related to fentanyl and its analogs; this is an increase from 55% in 2016. So, Canada also has its opioid crisis, albeit to a lesser degree than ours.[36]

The Centers for Disease Control and Prevention or CDC stated that in 2016, the number of fatal overdoses involving opioids was five times higher than in 1999. Also, between 1999 and 2016, the total deaths from drug overdoses were over 630,000. Sixty-six percent (66%) of these deaths, involved opioids. Approximately 40% of all opioid deaths involved **legal-prescription opioids** such as OxyContin or oxycodone, hydrocodone, and morphine. **Non-Prescription illegal opioids** such as heroin and **Illicitly Manufactured Fentanyl (IMF)** accounted for the majority of deaths resulting from illegal opioids.[3]

More than 42,000 people were killed in 2016 from all opioid overdoses. Comparing the years 2015 and 2016, overdose fatalities from IMF more than doubled from 9,580 to 19,413, respectively. For these same years, heroin deaths increased by nearly 19.5%, while that from legal painkillers increased by 10.6%.[4]

The problems caused by the opioid epidemic have not improved significantly. Overdose deaths from IMF are outpacing that of other illegal opioids by far as it becomes more available, cheaper, and deadlier.[5] In fact, over 72,000 people are estimated or projected to have died from drug-related overdoses in 2017 compared to more than 63,600 who died in 2016.[1,3,35]

The Human Health Services Acting Secretary declared a Public Health Emergency to address National Opioid Crisis in October 2017. [2]

In age-adjusted drug-overdose death rates, by opioid category:
United States, 1999 – 2016
SOURCE: NCHS, National Vital Statistics System, Mortality.

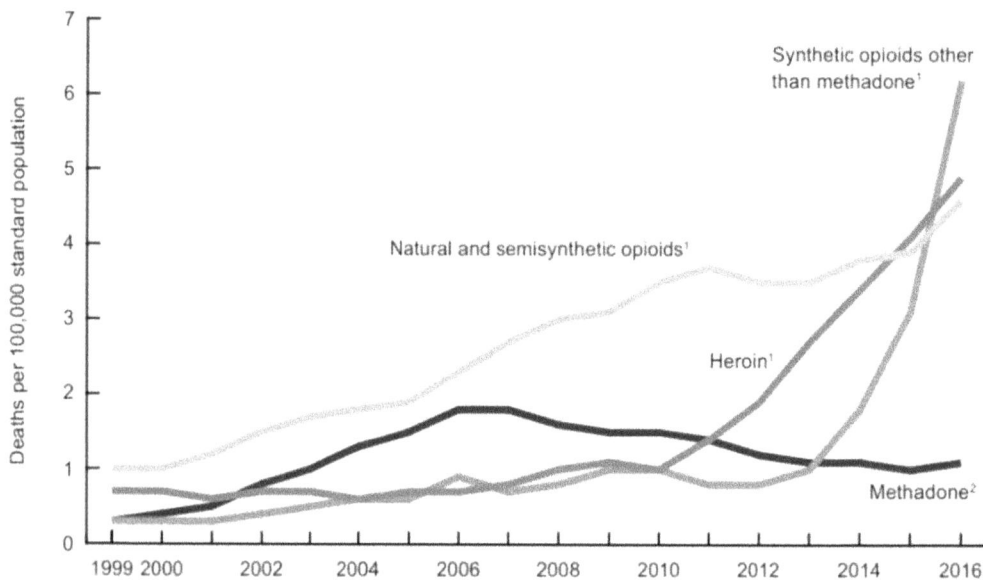

Note how fast the death rate climbed between 2014 and 2016 for synthetic opioids (such as IMF). This resulted in almost a straight upward line in 2016.[6] The projected or estimated number of deaths is even greater for 2017.[35]

A major contributing factor to the opioid epidemic is the **non-opioid drug-related overdose deaths** caused by drugs like **cocaine, methamphetamine, many other illegal drugs, and their analogs**. This category accounted for about 34% of the total drug-related overdose deaths in the United States in 2016.

What makes this category so important is that an ever- increasing number of opioid deaths are directly related to this class of drugs, hence compounding the problems of opioid drug overdoses. In addition, there are also legally prescribed drugs such as **benzodiazepines, other sedatives, and the overuse of alcohol**, which add to the existing problems.[1]

Despite increased awareness and efforts made to address the opioid epidemic, the CDC reports that between the third quarter of 2016 and the third quarter of 2017 (July 2016 through September 2017), opioid overdoses have increased by about 29.7%. This was documented by visits to emergency rooms and hospitals across the United States. The Midwest had 69.7%, followed by the West with 40.3%, Northeast with 21.3%, Southwest with 20.2%, and Southeast with a 14% increase.[7]

The figure below shows a consistent rise in deaths up to 2017 related to opioid overdose.

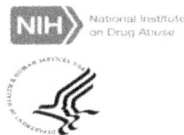

National Overdose Deaths—Number of Deaths Involving Opioid Drugs. *The figure above is a bar chart showing the total number of U.S. overdose deaths involving opioid drugs from 2002 to 2016, and provisional 2017 data. Included in this number are opioid analgesics, along with heroin and illicit synthetic opioids. The chart is overlaid by a line graph showing the number of deaths of females (top) and males (bottom) from 2002 to 2016. From 2002-2017, there was a 4.1-fold increase in the total number of deaths.*

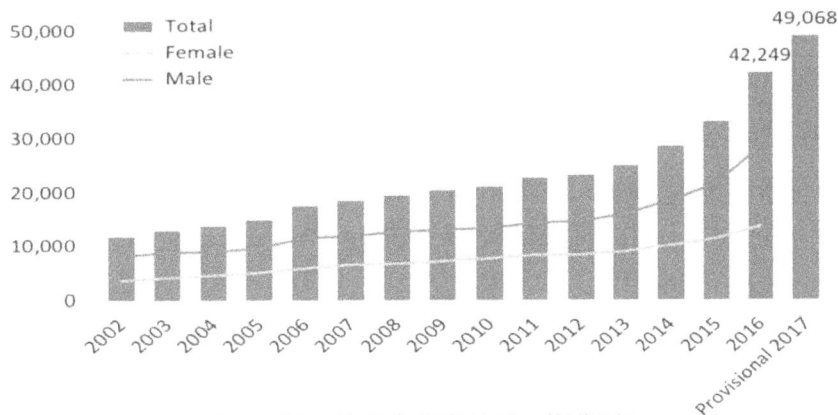

The economic costs will obviously continue to rise because of the increase in the number of deaths and opioid-related overdoses. In 2016, more than 42,000 people lost their lives to opioid-related overdoses; over 49,000 is expected in 2017 once the numbers are finalized.

The Economic Burden

The economic burden, including healthcare costs, continues to rise. In November 2017, the Council of Economic Advisers (CEA) reports that the estimated opioid- crisis costs were at $504 billion in 2015, when about 33,000 people lost their lives to opioid overdose. The CEA also estimated that in 2013, the cost was $78.5 billion, now considered a significant underestimation.[8,9]

How Did this Opioid Epidemic Start? Who Is Responsible?

The general belief is that the opioid epidemic is primarily a result of an ever-increasing number of legal opioid prescriptions. The CDC reports that the number of prescriptions quadrupled between 1999 and 2010. This caused an increased amount of dispensed oxycodone, hydrocodone, and morphine. Although the rise in prescriptions peaked in 2010, it still remains high but decreased by about 18% by 2015.

The amount of opioids prescribed in the United States peaked at 782 morphine milligram equivalents (MME) per capita (per person) in 2010, then decreased to 640 MME per capita in 2015. However, the deaths from opioid overdose, remained high and continued to rise from 1999, and was about five times what it was by 2016.[6] It is also worth noting that despite the overall decline in opioid prescriptions in the country, they were many cities that had an MME per capita of about 2000 in 2015.

For example, three cities in Virginia — Galax, Norton, and Martinsville — had MMEs ranging from over 3000 and to 4000 plus per capita in 2015. Hence, Virginia was one of the states with the highest number of overdoses and drug- related deaths in 2015.[6,13] The other significant factor contributing to drug overdose and deaths is illegal drugs such as heroin and IMF.

The opioid epidemic is said to have occurred in three waves. The first was in the 1990s and associated with the overprescription of opioids. The second occurred at about 2010, which saw a rapid increase in heroin-overdose deaths, and was also the peak of availability for opioid prescriptions. The third phase began around 2013 when IMF was used in combination with heroin to produce a more potent drug cocktail.[1]

The graph below shows that by the end of 2016, the number of deaths from IMF exceeded over 20,000, while heroin exceeded 15,000, and prescription opioids about 14,000. However, the most frightening aspect of this was a dramatic increase in IMF, from which deaths more than doubled compared to 2015 figures. Heroin deaths increased by about 20%, and legal prescription drug-related overdose deaths increased by about 10.6%.[4]

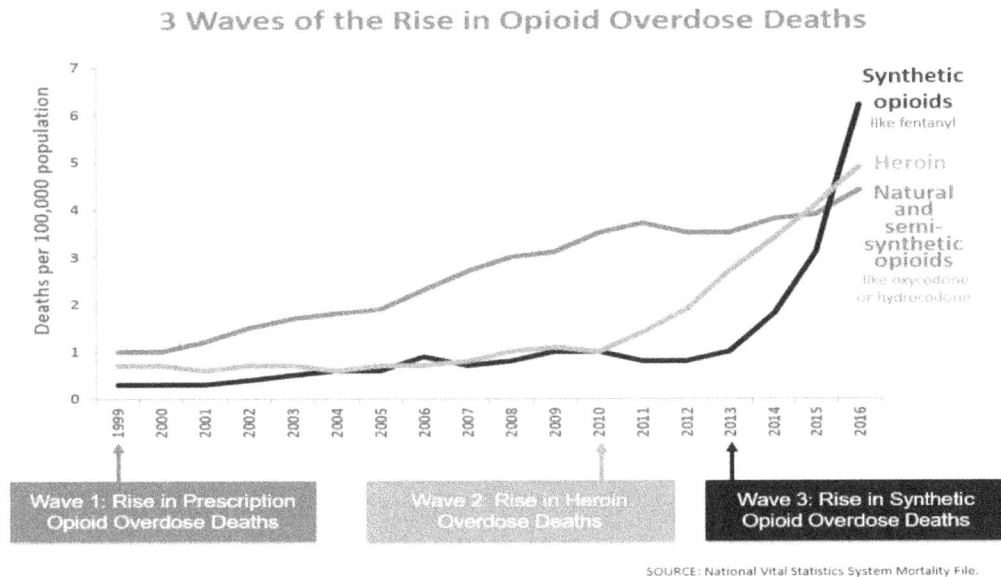

3 Waves of the Rise in Opioid Overdose Deaths

SOURCE: National Vital Statistics System Mortality File.

Let's be clear: although the opioid epidemic is now front and center of our healthcare and economic crises, this did not just start in the 1990s, or with doctors prescribing more opioids than what was prescribed before. Do you know that:

The U.S. has a long history of drug abuse. Legally, the United States imported opium for more than a hundred years. Morphine was in common use during the Civil War. Heroin was manufactured by the end of the nineteenth century. and cocaine, long a popular tonic, was marketed as a cure for narcotic addiction? [11]

In 1907, the US estimated that its population was at 87 million people, and about 200,000 were estimated to be addicted to opioids.[14] In 1906, the Pure Food and Drug Act was passed, in part requiring better labeling for medications, including opioids and even cocaine.[15] Now things are getting out of control, and a significant number of people are dying at an alarming rate from overdoses of opioids and other illegal drugs, so we are confronted with an opioid epidemic.

No Specific Government or Politician or Their Administration is Exempt

It is also important to realize that no specific government or politician or their administration is exempt from being blame for the opioid epidemic; or was totally unaware of drug abuse, drug use, and the potential of a drug or an opioid epidemic. Numerous bills have been passed, and some of them were subsequently amended by different administrations. In addition, there have been various policies put in place. New rules have also been enacted at both federal and state level. Here is a very small sample of some of them; this is not a complete representation of what each administration and its listed president have done:

Pres. Abraham Lincoln[31] speaking about alcoholics on February 24, 1842:

> In my judgment, such of us as have never fallen victims, have been spared more from the absence of appetite, than from any mental or moral superiority over those who have.

The Pure Food and Drug Act was passed in 1906 by Pres. Theodore Roosevelt, Jr.[15] The Harrison Narcotics Tax Act of 1914 was a United States federal law that regulated and taxed the production, importation, and distribution of opiates and coca products. It was signed by Pres. Woodrow Wilson[11,12] on December 17, 1914.

Pres. Lyndon B. Johnson's[33] remarks at the signing of the Drug Abuse Control Amendments Bill on July 15, 1965:

> Drugs can, if properly used, protect our health, prolong our life, reduce much pain and suffering. Improperly used, drugs can cause great injury and do great harm.

> The Drug Abuse Control Act of 1965 is designed to prevent both the misuse and the illicit traffic of potentially dangerous drugs, especially the sedatives and the stimulants, which are so important in the medicines that we use today.

The Comprehensive Drug Abuse Prevention and Control Act/The Controlled Substance Act of 1970 regulated in part the manufacturer position and/or trafficking of drugs/substances. It was signed by Pres. Richard Nixon on October 27, 1970.

Pres. Gerald R. Ford's[34] Statement on Actions to Congress to Combat Drug Abuse, December 26, 1975:

Drug abuse is a tragic national problem which saps our Nation's vitality. It is also a major contributor to our growing crime rate. All of us must redouble our efforts to combat this problem.

Pres. Jimmy Carter: Drug Abuse Message to Congress, August 2, 1977

My goals are to discourage all drug abuse in America—and also discourage the excessive use of alcohol and tobacco—and to reduce to a minimum the harm drug abuse causes when it does occur.

Pres. Carter endorses decriminalization of marijuana.[17]

Anti-Drug Abuse Act of 1986

Pres. Ronald Reagan[18] created the Office of National Drug Control Policy in 1988. Its director (drug czar) was responsible for coordinating activities related to drugs such as healthcare, legislative research, and governmental issues.

First Lady Nancy Reagan was also known for her "just say no" anti-drug message.

Pres. George H.W. Bush (Sr.): Address to the Nation on the National Drug Control Strategy, September 5, 1989[19]

This is the first time since taking the oath of office that I felt an issue was so important, so threatening, that it warranted talking directly with you, the American people. All of us agree that the gravest domestic threat facing our nation today is drugs. Drugs have strained our faith in our system of justice. Our courts, our prisons, our legal system, are stretched to the breaking point.

Pres. Bill Clinton elevated the director's position at the Office of National Drug Control Policy to Cabinet-level in 1993 - Drug Czar. His "three strikes" crime bill was passed in 1994, at the height of the crack cocaine epidemic.[21]

Pres. George W. Bush: Bush Announces Drug Control Strategy, February12, 2002[20]

> We've got a problem in this country. Too many people use drugs, and this is an individual tragedy. And, as a result, it is a social crisis. There is no question that drug use wreaks havoc on the very fabric that provides stability for our society. Drug use wreaks havoc on our families. Drug use destroys people's ambitions and hopes.

The Secure and Responsible Drug Disposal Act of 2010, also called the Disposal Act.

Recovery Enhancement for Addiction Treatment Act or the TREAT Act. (Sec.2) This bill amends the Controlled Substances Act to revise the requirements for a practitioner to administer, dispense, or prescribe narcotic drugs for maintenance or detoxification treatment in an office-based opioid treatment program. April 27, 2016.

Pres. Barack Obama[22,32]

H.R. 6, Substance Use-Disorder Prevention that Promotes Opioid Recovery and Treatment (SUPPORT) for Patients and Communities Act, June 22, 2018.

Statement of Declaration: The Human Health Services Acting Secretary declared a Public Health Emergency to Address National Opioid Crisis in October 2017.

The President's Commission on Combating Drug Addiction and Opioid Crisis.

Pres. Donald Trump [2,23,38]

The Pharmaceutical Companies' Role

The increase in the availability of prescription drugs to patients is also believed to be partly attributable to major pharmaceutical companies that promoted and marketed opioids as drugs with minimum addictive potential and significant benefits for reducing pain. Drug companies had vigorous advertising campaigns, utilizing all media with print advertisements, infomercials, and short commercials.[24,25] There have been many lawsuits, sanctions, findings and still-pending litigation against pharmaceutical companies for the role that they are believed to have played in this opioid epidemic.

The Veterans Health Administration

In 2000, the Veterans Health Administration or VHA established a new protocol for patients under their care. It included "pain as the fifth vital sign" along with blood pressure, heart rate, respiration, and temperature. This resulted in more attention being paid to patients with pain and providing treatments for them with opioids as well as other medications.[26]

The Federal Government's Role

Every drug that is approved in the United States of America has to go through very rigorous scientific process and other protocols. The DEA and the FDA in part are ultimately responsible for all drugs that are approved for use by the consumers and for research purposes. It is well documented that pharmaceutical companies played a role in the opioid epidemic as did medical doctors and providers. It must also be noted that the DEA, FDA and by extension the federal government also had a pivotal role in their assessment, evaluation and approval of opioids.

These opioids were associated with the "beginning of the opioid epidemic" when oxycontin was king. They continue to play a pivotal role in the current opioid epidemic. Also, one cannot forget the strong support given to pharmaceutical companies by some members of the Senate as well as Congress which effectively empowered these companies as well as creating a climate where approval of opioids from the DEA/FDA were easy to be obtained. In return, the politicians were well compensated significantly by campaign contributions /other things that were given to them or their associates by pharmaceutical companies.[24,25]

Doctors and Healthcare Providers at a Crossroad

Doctors and healthcare providers were expected to address pain aggressively or face possible consequences, either from their State Medical Board or patients. For example, a physician was disciplined by the Oregon Medical Board in 1999 for not providing a satisfactory amount of pain medication for six patients.[27] And in California, a jury found a physician guilty of committing elderly abuse by not adequately treating the patient's pain. That case resulted from a lawsuit against the physician in 2001.[28]

As a result of these and other pressures, as well as aggressive promotion by pharmaceutical companies and the medical establishment, the prescribers of opioids were at a crossroads and opted to escalate opioid prescriptions.[25]

In our current climate, the pendulum has swung the opposite way. Now, physicians and opioid prescribers are afraid of prescribing opioids because of the potential risk of going to jail or being disciplined, even for what may be considered legitimate use. Of course, there are illegal acts by and unethical conduct from some physicians/medical providers who prescribed opioids.[29,30]

References, Recommended Readings and Resources

1. Centers for Disease Control and Prevention. Understanding the Epidemic. https://www.cdc.gov/drugoverdose/epidemic/index.html. Last visited June 16, 2018.
2. HHS Acting Secretary Declares Public Health Emergency to Address National Opioid Crisis. https://www.hhs.gov/about/news/2017/10/26/ hhs-acting-secretary-declares-public-health-emergency-address- national-opioid-crisis.html. Accessed March 7, 2018.
3. Provisional Drug Overdose Death Counts 12 Month-ending Provisional Number of Drug Overdose. Deaths. Based on data available for analysts. June 3, 2018. https://www.cdc.gov/nchs/nvss/ vsrr/drug-overdose-data.htm. Last accessed June 23, 2018.
4. Puja Seth, Ph.D.; Lawrence Scholl, Ph.D.; Rose A. Rudd, MSPH; Sarah Bacon, Ph.D., *MMMWR*. Overdose deaths involving opioids, cocaine, and psychostimulants – United States, 2015 – 2016. https:// www.cdc.gov/mmwr/volumes/67/wr/mm6712a1.htm. Accessed May 5, 2018.
5. Gery P. Guy Jr., Ph.D.; Kun Zhang, Ph.D.; Michele K. Bohm, MPH; Jan Losby, Ph.D.;

   Brian Lewis; Randall Young, MA; Louise B. Murphy, Ph.D.; Deborah Dowell, MD· CDCMMWR. Vital Signs: Changes in Opioid Prescribing in the United States, 2006–2015. July 7, 2017 / 66(26);697-704. https://www.cdc.gov/mmwr/volumes/66/wr/ mm6626a4.htm?s_cid=mm6626a4_w. Accessed March 1, 2018.
6. U.S. drug overdose deaths continue to rise; increase fueled by synthetic opioids. https://www.cdc.gov/media/releases/2018/p0329- drug-overdose-deaths.html. Accessed May 5th, 2018.
7. Alana M. Vivolo-Kantor, Ph.D.; Puja Seth, Ph.D.; R. Matthew Gladden, Ph.D.; Christine L. Mattson, Ph.D.; Grant T. Baldwin, Ph.D.; Aaron Kite-Powell, MS; Michael A. Coletta, MPH Vital Signs: Trends in Emergency Department Visits for Suspected Opioid Overdoses — United States, July 2016–September 2017 *March 6, 2018,* MMWR.https://www.cdc.gov/mmwr/volumes/67/wr/mm6709e1.htm. Accessed June 17, 2018.
8. The Underestimated Cost of the Opioid Crisis. The Economic Advisory Council November 2017. https://www.whitehouse.gov/sites/ whitehouse.gov/files/images/The%20Underestimated%20Cost%20 of%20the%20Opioid%20Crisis.pdf. Accessed June 15, 2018.
9. NIH. National Institute on Drug Abuse. Opioid overdose Crisis. https://www.drugabuse.gov/drugs-abuse/opioids/opioid-overdose- crisis. Accessed June 4, 2018.
10. Drug Enforcement Administration. Drug Facts Sheet-Narcotics. https://www.dea.gov/druginfo/drug_data_sheets/Narcotics.pdf. Accessed July 4, 2018.
11. Drug Enforcement Administration (DEA) The Early Years. https:// www.dea.gov/sites/default/files/2018-05/Early%20Years%20p%2012- 29.pdf Accessed July 23, 2018.

12. Harrison Narcotics Tax Act of 1914: Pres. Woodrow Wilson. December 17, 1914, https://en.wikipedia.org/wiki/War_on_drugs. Last accessed July 23, 2018.

13. National Opioid Epidemic. amfAR, Opioid, and Healthcare Indicated Database. http://opioid.amfar.org/indicator/mme_percap. Accessed June 17, 2018.

14. Nick Stockton; Americans Have Been Addicted to Prescription Opiates Forever. 03.16.16. https://www.wired.com/2016/03/ Americans-addicted-prescription-opiates-forever/. Accessed June 17, 2018.

15. Pure Food and Drug Act (1906). https://www.encyclopedia.com/ history/united-states-and-canada/us-history/food-and-drug-act-1906. Accessed June 17, 2018.

16. Pres. Jimmy Carter drug abuse message to Congress, August 2, 1977. http://www.presidency.ucsb.edu/ws/?pid=7908. Accessed July 22, 2018.

17. Edward Walsh. Carter Endorses Decriminalization of Marijuana. August 3, 1977. https://www.washingtonpost.com/archive/ politics/1977/08/03/carter-endorsesecriminalization-of-marijuana/7e. Accessed July 22, 2018.

18. H.R.5484 - Anti-Drug Abuse Act of 1986. October 27, 1986. https:// www.congress.gov/bill/99th-congress/house-bill/5484. Accessed July 22, 2018.

19. Pres. George H Bush. Address to the Nation on the National Drug Control Strategy. September 5, 1989. http://www.presidency.ucsb.edu/ ws/?pid=17472. Accessed July 22, 2018.

20. President George W. Bush. Bush Announces Drug Control Strategy. February 12, 2002. https://2001-2009.state.gov/p/inl/rls/rm/8451.htm. Accessed July 22, 2018.

21. BBC News US and Canada, Bill Clinton regrets 'three strikes' bill. July 16, 2015. https://www.bbc.com/news/world-us-canada-33545971. Accessed July 22, 2018.

22. S.1455 - TREAT Act. Recovery Enhancements for Addiction Treatment Act April 27, 2016, https://www.congress.gov/bill/114th- congress/senate-bill/1455. Last visited July 22, 2018.

23. H.R. 6, Substance Use-Disorder Prevention that Promotes Opioid Recovery and Treatment (SUPPORT) for Patients and Communities Act. June 22, 2018. https://policy.house.gov/legislative/bills/hr-6- substance-use-disorder-prevention-promotes-opioid-recovery-and- treatment. Accessed June 23, 2018.

24. Harvard Study: Big Pharma, US Gov. Behind Opioid Epidemic. July 27, 2017, Sean Adl-Tabatabai News, US 105. https://yournewswire. com/harvard-study-opioid-epidemic/. Accessed March 12, 2018.

25. Richie Farrell. The Opioid Epidemic: How Big Pharma and Congress Created America's Worst Health Crisis. 10/16/2017. https://www. huffingtonpost.com/entry/the-opioid-epidemic-how-big-pharma-and- congress-created_us_59e4e02ee4b003f928d5e8bf. Accessed March 7, 2018.

26. Department of Veterans Affairs, Pain as the Fifth Vital Sign Toolkit (October 2000) http://www.va.gov/PAINMANAGEMENT/docs/ TOOLKIT.pdf. Accessed March 10, 2018.

27. Oregon Board Disciplines Doctor for Not Treating Patients' Pain," New York Times, September 4, 1999. http://www.nytimes.com/1999/09/04/us/oregon-board-disciplines-doctor-for-not-treating- patients-pain.html. Accessed March 10, 2018.

28. Bergman v. Eden Medical Center, No. H205732-1 (Cal. Super. Ct., Alameda County, 2001). https://www.highbeam.com/ doc/1G1-79341880.html. Accessed March 10, 2018.

29. Furrow, B. R. "Pain Management and Provider Liability: No More Excuses" Journal of Law, Medicine & Ethics 29, no. 1(2001): 28– 51, SAGE Journals. http://journals.sagepub.com/doi/10.1111/j.1748- 720X.2001.tb00038.x. Accessed March 10, 2018.

30. Perry G Fine, West J Med… Fear, and Loathing on the Care Path Treating Pain and Suffering. 2002 Jan; 176(1):17. https://www.ncbi. nlm.nih.gov/pmc/articles/PMC1071643/. Accessed March 10, 2018.

31. Pres. Abraham Lincoln on Addiction. From the Collected Works of Abraham Lincoln. Rutgers University Press, 1953, the Abraham Lincoln Association, Roy P. Basler, Ed. http://www.dpft.org/lincoln. htm. Accessed July 23, 2018.

32. Secure and Responsible Drug Disposal Act of 2009. S. 1292 (111th) https://www.govtrack.us/congress/bills/111/s1292 Accessed October22,1018.

33. Pres. Lyndon B. Johnson. Remarks at the Signing of the Drug Abuse Control Amendments Bill. - Address to Congress. July 15, 1965. http://www.presidency.ucsb.edu/ws/index.php?pid=27087. Last visited July 23, 2018.

34. Pres. Gerald R. Ford: Statement on Actions to Congress to Combat Drug Abuse. December 26, 1975. http://www.presidency.ucsb.edu/ws/ index.php?pid=5458. Accessed July 23, 2018.

35. NIH. National Institute of Drug Abuse. Overdose Death Rates Revised August 2018. https://www.drugabuse.gov/related-topics/trends- statistics/overdose-death-rates. Accessed August 16, 2018.

36. National report: Apparent opioid-related deaths in Canada. (released June 2018). https://www.canada.ca/en/public-health/services/ publications/healthy-living/national-report-apparent-opioid-related- deaths-released-june-2018.html. Last visited August 19, 2018.

37. Keith Humphreys. Americans use far more opioids than anyone else in the world. March 5, 2017. https://www.washingtonpost.com/news/ wonk/wp/2017/03/15/americans-use-far-more-opioids-than-anyone- else-in-the-world/?utm_term=.be634a22752e. Accessed August 19, 2018.

38. The President's Commission on Combating Drug Addiction and Opioid Crisis. March 29, 2017, https://www.whitehouse.gov/sites/whitehouse.gov/files/images/Final_ Report_Draft_11-1-2017.pdf Accessed August

Chapter 2

"Lock Them Up, Those Pain Doctors……!!!!"

Who is a Pain Doctor?

Pain management or pain medicine doctors, sometimes referred to as interventional pain doctors are medical providers who most often are board-certified, board-eligible or appropriately credentialed in the discipline/specialty of pain medicine to manage and treat patients with pain. They may have their primary board certification in physical medicine and rehabilitation, anesthesiology, neurology, psychiatry and, to a lesser degree, radiology.[1,2] After attaining board certification in their primary specialty, they earn certification in pain management, pain medicine or interventional pain management.

A few other major specialties also have providers with pain management board certifications. These providers take a comprehensive approach to the management of pain by utilizing and collaborating with other services or disciplines. These include, but are not limited to: physical therapy, occupational therapy, massage therapy, chiropractic care, cognitive behavioral therapy, biofeedback, interventional pain procedures, medications, and psychotherapy.

We often work with many consultants/physicians and medical providers to facilitate appropriate care for each patient.[3] The management of a significant number of patients seen by pain-management consultants or providers requires a multidisciplinary approach. This becomes even more important for patients who require chronic opioid treatment and have significant comorbidities such as psychiatric disorders, pulmonary disease, renal disease, and liver disorder.

Who is NOT a Pain Doctor?

All doctors who have a medical license are generally licensed by the state in which they are working to practice medicine and perform surgery. The practice of medicine in each state includes (but is not limited to) prescribing numerous medications with exceptions that generally include opioids and other controlled substances. These exceptions are addressed by the DEA that grants licenses to prescribe opioids and controlled substances. Not all medical doctors/providers are licensed or authorized to prescribe.

The DEA credentials doctors/providers they deem appropriate for different levels of eligibility for writing prescriptions. Most doctors/providers, regardless of their primary specialties and subspecialties, are eligible to prescribe most opioids typically used to treat most patients requiring pain medications. This means that family practice physicians, internal medicine doctors, pediatricians, endocrinologists, infectious disease doctors or pulmonologists, dentists, and podiatrists (to name a few) are likely to have the same or a very similar writing privilege for opioids as the physicians/providers that are board-certified in pain management.

Now this, of course, does not mean that they will all go out and start writing prescriptions for opioids in quantities similar to that of pain management specialists. However, some do. The reality is that most physicians/providers don't and probably will never do it. However, those that sometimes did their actions resulted in the rise and proliferation of the **'Pill mills.'** These are essentially medical clinics in which the medical doctors, clinic providers or pharmacists prescribed and or dispense opioids or control substances illegitimately for presumed medical purposes. Usually cash for services.

The doctors and providers associated with these clinics are from many different specialties, they prescribe in general large quantities of opioids and controlled substances, ultimately resulting in the overprescription of these drugs. In some instances, some of these providers were prescribing far more opioids than probably most pain management specialists would consider doing.

The pain doctor is **<u>NOT</u>** a doctor who simply prescribes narcotics or opioids to patients who present to them with pain. There are several providers who have taken this approach, although not necessarily under the umbrella of pain management. Some are primary care physicians, associated mid-level providers, or members of different specialties.

I believe the vast majority of them are doing an excellent job of trying to treat their patients' conditions and taking the necessary steps to do so while using opioids.

However, there is a significant number of healthcare providers who have failed to meet the minimum standards required to treat patients requesting opioids or who are in need of opioids to manage what is referred to as pain or pain-related conditions. This has led to the emergence of a group of doctors, providers, and businessmen who have created the aforementioned pill mills.

The concept of the Pill mill seems to have evolved and grown in parallel with the increase in pain prescriptions for opioids and other controlled substances, from about the late 1990s and becoming more significant around 2010. The state of Florida, for example, had a significant number of Pill mills. Providers, doctors, and mid-levels in the state were reported as prescribing and/or dispensing the largest amount of narcotics/opioids in the country, which was higher than all the other states combined. The 'OxyContin Express' or 'Oxy Express' was related to the overprescription of OxyContin/oxycodone and other controlled substances during the peak years of pill mill operations.[4,5,6,7]

Florida then enacted legislation that would govern and dictate the operation of pain clinics, referred to as the Pill mill Laws. Many other states have since done the same. Although there are differences between the various states' laws, there are certain features that are usually held in common. These may include, but are not limited to the following:

➢ Each clinic must be owned by a physician who is licensed or trained, in the practice of pain medicine or appropriately credentialed, therefore eliminating the businessman who typically funds these clinics.

➢ These clinics would be limited to dispensing opioids from their offices unless they are registered with their State's Pharmacy Board and or State Medical Board as well as meeting other criteria.

➢ Clinics treating more than 50% of its patients as pain management patients with Schedule II - III controlled substances/opioids (see Appendix B) must be registered, and part of its practice's name must include the word 'pain.' Their patients must be properly assessed to determine if they are appropriate for pain management before the start of treatment. If they meet the criteria for acute or chronic pain management, they must be properly monitored continuously by the providers for subsequent visits. Failure to comply with the law may lead to a felony conviction. No one with a felony conviction would be granted a license to operate or be the owner of a pain clinic.

Since the law was enacted in Florida, significant improvements have been noted concerning opioid prescriptions and the divergence of opioids. This also led to a considerable reduction in overdoses and deaths related to opioids use, as well as to other illegal drugs. Another factor which has led to a significant reduction in Pill mills and doctor-shopping is the creation of a state database, the **Prescription Drug Monitoring Program** or PDMP. This partly allows physicians and providers to identify patients who are obtaining prescriptions from multiple providers.

Florida is now considered safer since the implementation of the Pill mill Laws and its state's PDMP. Significant progress has been made in Florida as well as other states, but there is still much more to be done regarding the opioid epidemic. Florida is no longer the state with the highest opioid prescriptions; according to the CDC in 2016, the five states with the highest rate of fatal overdose were West Virginia (52.0 per 100,000), Ohio (39.1 per 100,000), New Hampshire (39.0 per 100,000), Pennsylvania (37.9 per 100,000), and Kentucky (33.5 per 100,000).[8] Also according to the CDC, overdoses increased by 30% from July 2016 to September 2017 in 52 areas in 45 states.[10]

Looking at the Evidence Against Pain Doctors

Prescription opioids are considered the primary reason for the opioid epidemic. The CDC stated that between 1999 and 2010, prescription opioids quadrupled and peaked in 2010.[15] The opioid-overdose deaths closely parallel the increase in legally prescribed opioids, which continued to decline after the year 2010.

In 2016, the total number of deaths (over 42,000) involving opioids, such as legal prescription opioids, illegal opioids, IMF, and heroin, was five times higher than in 1999.[11,17]

However, by 2016, opioid prescriptions declined by about 18%, although opioid-related deaths continued to increase. By the year 2015, the number of opioid prescriptions declined to about three times what they were in 1999.[15] Opioid prescription-related deaths from 2002 to 2011 saw a twofold increase.

Since 2011, deaths related to opioid prescriptions, although with minor decreases, have remained relatively stable.[18]

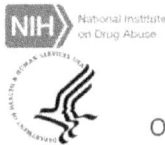

National Overdose Deaths
Number of Deaths Involving
Opioid Pain Relievers (excluding non-methadone synthetics)

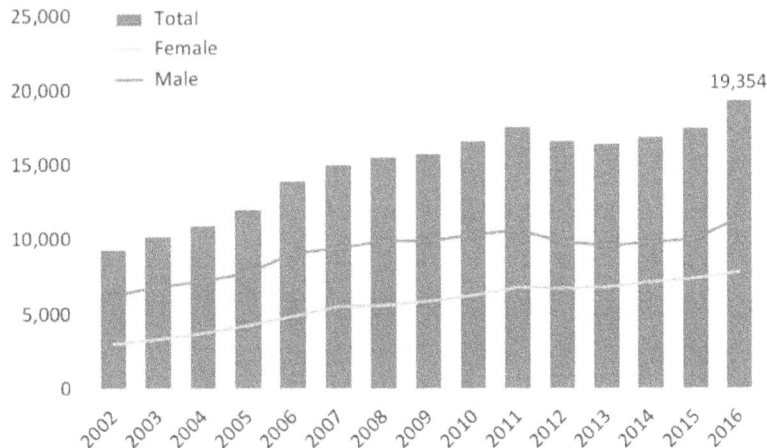

National Overdose Deaths—Number of Deaths Involving Prescription Opioid Pain Relievers (excluding non-methadone synthetics). *The figure above is a bar chart showing the total number of U.S. overdose deaths involving opioid pain relievers (excluding non-methadone synthetics) from 2002 to 2016. Non-methadone synthetics is a category dominated by illicit fentanyl and has been excluded to more accurately reflect deaths from prescription opioids. The chart is overlaid by a line graph showing the number of deaths of females (bottom line) and males (top line). From 2002 to 2011, there was a 1.9-fold increase in the total number of deaths, but it has remained relatively stable since then.[18]*

The total number of opioid-related deaths is about 66% of all drug overdose- related deaths. Approximately 60% of this number is related to non- prescription opioids such as that from illegal heroin and manufactured illegal fentanyl, and 40% is related to legal prescription opioids such as oxycodone, hydrocodone and morphine.[11,17]

Of course, another way of saying this is: of all the drug-overdose deaths in the United States, about 26% is directly attributed to prescription-related opioids, about 40% is related to illegal opioid drugs such as heroin and IMF, and about 34% is related to drug overdoses not primarily from opioids. However, if stated this way, it may oversimplify the gravity of the situation and probably take away the focus from an area (in this case, prescription drugs) that has seen more increase than any of the other two categories over the same period.

Prescription drugs are under attack because of the belief and evidence that this may directly lead to, or at the very least, contribute to the increase of illegal opioid use and overdose deaths. The argument often made is that there would be less demand for illegal opioids once fewer patients are using less prescription opioids resulting in fewer of them becoming addicted to their legal prescriptions. On the other hand, it is not unreasonable or irrational to say that if there were no illegal opioids such as heroin or manufactured fentanyl, that the 40% who died from an illegal opioid overdose would be significantly less. The deaths from the withdrawal of legal opioids pale in comparison to that from illegal opioids or illegal drugs in general.

Having made these points do not negate the importance of responsible opioid prescriptions or the need for legislation such as the Pill mill Laws and others. This law has or has had very little adverse or no effect on the way the vast majority of legitimate pain clinics operate.

The primary reason for that is most of the clinics that previously operated as pain clinics were doing the things that the law required before it was changed. Probably in most instances, the most difficult part of this process was filling out the application to be a licensed pain clinic. Even for most primary care physicians, family doctors or internal medicine physicians, and those with subspecialties like orthopedic doctors, dentists, general surgeons and podiatrists, the law did not have a significant negative impact on the way they practice.

The classic example is the patient who presents to a legitimate pain clinic on high-dose opioids: greater than a 100-milligram MME daily dose. Sometimes, these patients are on several hundred MME/day referred from wherever, and they expect to "have refills and continue medicating the way they are used to getting it" because their primary care doctors gave them just enough opioids to last until they see the new pain management doctor. The patients then discover that the process involves, but is not limited to: their medical records looked at and reviewed in detail, providing their medical history, providing or obtaining diagnostic studies, completing a physical examination, and giving urine or oral sample for testing.

The patients may also be surprised to know that there is no guarantee they will walk out with any medications at all. They will also realize that although it is important, their current medications may not determine what their next narcotic/ opioid prescriptions will ultimately be. Patients like these may be seen once and may not return because the requirements of the legitimate pain clinic ask for more than what they are willing to comply with.

The same patients may walk into a Pill mill and walk out with more medications than they previously took, with only a cursory attempt of an evaluation/assessment of their medical condition if they are willing to pay in cash.

Alternatively, they could walk into non-pain specialist clinics who are legitimately practicing and have no intention of breaking the laws; in some cases, they may leave with medications comparable to what they would get from the Pill mills. For this group of physicians as well as other physicians/providers, the CDC guidelines of 2016 for opioid prescriptions may be of significant benefit.[11]

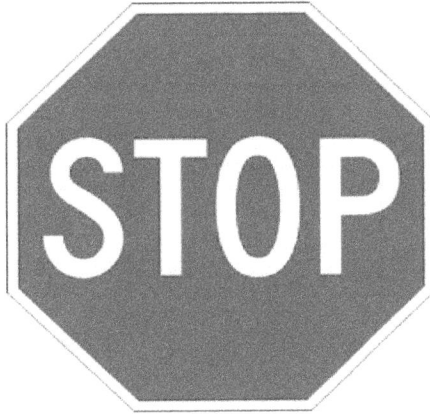

Breaking News: Pain Management Doctors are Responsible for <u>Less than Six</u> <u>(6) %</u> of All the Opioid Prescriptions Written in the United States

If I were to say to you that there were a lot of opioids prescribed in this country that have contributed to the opioid epidemic, and that pain management doctors are responsible for the epidemic, these two statements would probably make sense to a significant number of people, even for professionals who work in pain management and addiction medicine. Unfortunately, most medical professionals and the public at large have failed to understand the role of pain management providers.

In an article published in the *American Journal of Preventive Medicine* in September 2015, the authors looked at how dentists, not pain management doctors, compared with other specialties in prescribing opioids.

This article's methodology or support material has nothing to do with pain management or pain management associations. The article's timing is important in that it covers the period from 2007 to 2012. This includes the year 2010, which CDC stated was the peak year of opioid prescriptions in the United States.[14,15]

The authors found the data as shown in the following table and figure. The table was modified in this book to include the category "**Opioid Prescription Percent**" using the same data they provided.[15]

Opioid Prescription Table

Specialty	Opioid Prescription (millions)	Opioid Prescription Percent (%)	Total Prescriptions (millions)	Opioid Prescribing Rate (%)
Pain Medicine	*14.5*	*5.02*	*29.8*	*48.7*
Surgery	28.3	9.80	77.6	36.5
Physical Medicine and Rehab	9.3	3.22	26.1	35.6
Dentistry	**18.5**	**6.40**	**64**	**28.9**
Emergency Medicine	12.5	4.33	60.5	20.7
General Practice	32.2	11.15	431.2	7.5
Non-Physician Prescriber	32.2	11.15	447.3	7.2
Family Practice	52.5	18.17	946.9	5.5
Internal Medicine	43.6	15.09	913.9	4.8
All Others	45.3	15.68	1252	3.6
Total	288.9	**100.00**	4191.7	100

Notes

"Non-physician prescribers" include nurse practitioners and physician assistants. "General practice" includes specialists in osteopathic medicine, general practice, and preventive medicine.

"Surgery" includes specialists in general, orthopedic, plastic, cardiothoracic, vascular, colorectal, spinal and neurologic surgery. "All others" includes specialists in cardiology, critical care, dermatology, endocrinology, gastroenterology, geriatrics, hematology, infectious disease, neurology, obstetrics and gynecology, oncology, otolaryngology, palliative care, pathology, pediatrics, podiatry, psychiatry, pulmonology, radiology, rheumatology, urology, and veterinary

Source: American Journal of Preventive Medicine (with permission).

Opioid Prescription (%)

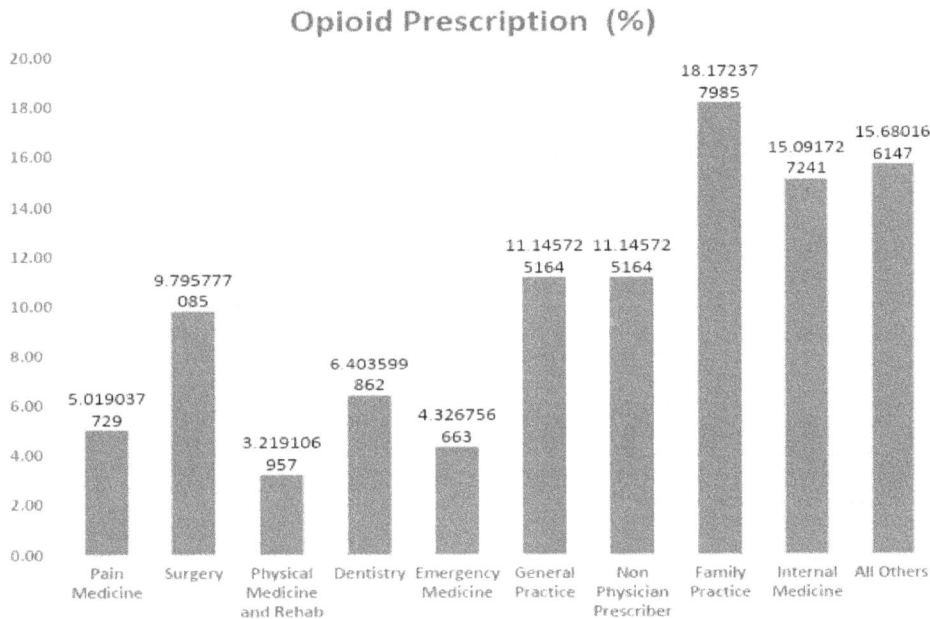

Clearly, it shows that even dentists write more opioid prescriptions than pain management doctors. You can also see that **pain management specialists do not write more than 94% of all the opioid prescriptions in this country**. However, most articles that described this study and others have focused on the Opioid Prescribing Rate, "which in this article shows pain management or pain medicine at 48.7%."

So, what does that mean? Simply, it means that for all the prescriptions written by pain medicine practitioners, a little less than half are opioids. The others may include but are not limited to anti-inflammatory, muscle relaxers, neuropathic medications, etc.

The CDC summarizes the article this way:

> *The supply of prescription opioids remains high in the U.S. An estimated 1 out of 5 patients with non-cancer pain or pain-related diagnoses are prescribed opioids in office-based settings. From 2007 – 2012, the rate of opioid prescribing has steadily increased among specialists more likely to manage acute and chronic pain. Prescribing rates are highest among pain medicine (49%), surgery (37%), and physical medicine/rehabilitation (36%). However, primary care providers account for about half of opioid pain relievers dispensed.*[16]

What was not said is that of all the prescriptions that were written, those three groups — pain medicine, physical medicine and rehab, and surgery — were responsible for only about 18% of the United States total. Alternatively, 82% of the prescriptions were written by providers other than members of those three groups. The question then becomes: why is that so bad? If I were to say to you that cardiothoracic surgeons perform more than 90% of the open-heart surgeries of the total surgeries they performed; endocrinologists who treat diabetes prescribed insulin and other diabetic medications for more than 50% of the total prescriptions; or infectious disease doctors prescribed antibiotics for more than 75% of their total prescriptions, would you think these are bad doctors or providers?

In fact, one may expect that both infectious disease and endocrinologists' providers/doctors will prescribe medications to treat infectious diseases and diabetes, respectively, at significantly higher rates than other doctors/providers. One could also expect that because there are so few infectious disease doctors and endocrinologists, the percentage of prescriptions they write will be minor compared to that of other doctors/providers. Just like almost any doctor/provider can write for pain management, so can most doctors write prescriptions for antibiotics and/ or diabetic medications. Of course, one would not expect other doctors to go around performing cardiothoracic surgeries, as this is a special skill requiring specific training and credentialing.

Therefore, expect the cardiothoracic surgeon to have an extremely high rate of specialty-specific procedures.

So, what happened with pain management doctors? Is there a reason why it is not expected that those of us who are pain management doctors have a higher percentage of our total prescriptions being opioids? Don't be alarmed by the "high prescription rate" of pain management doctors. It is the expectation that providers/ doctors who have specializations will utilize treatments for the areas in which they specialize more than other doctors/providers do in general. In fact, using the same numbers from this study that the CDC uses, if you grouped pain medicine, rehab medicine, surgery, dentistry, and emergency medicine, the average prescription rate for them is about 34%. Clearly, you can say that's very high. However, it is also worth considering the patient population these groups treat. Bear in mind that those groups of providers prescribed less than 30% of all the opioids prescribed in the United States.

The remaining medical providers prescribed more than 70% of the country's opioid prescriptions. However, they have an average prescription rate of about 5%, a very attractive number.

Some of you may cheer for this. But more than 70% of all the opioids that are out there, and for the most part are poorly monitored or not monitored at all, are coming from this group. Opioids are generally prescribed by providers who genuinely care about their patients, but often fail to properly monitor their opioids or controlled substance use, which is very dangerous, to say the least.

There is, of course, an argument that can be made. In the group of pain practice (or other practices), those of us who are in pain management, if there are pain management providers who were significantly outside of the normal range/average, then that needs to be addressed according to the specifics of those providers' practice. If someone is in pain management in general, and he or she has a prescribing rate of more than 90% (random percentage) for opioids out of his or her total prescriptions, and the average is 48.7% in the specialty, that needs to be addressed in context.

One very important point of this is:

you could take away or close all the pain management practices that currently exist in America today, and we would still have more than 94% of the prescriptions written by the other prescribers

I do not doubt that those patients who then would have no pain management providers would simply find their way back to the less-talked- about 94% providers.

Appropriately trained pain management specialists can and do make invaluable contributions in helping to curtail the opioid epidemic. As long as we stop confusing the writing of opioid prescriptions as equivalent to being pain management specialists, this terrible epidemic will have more than credible opponents as we all come together in fighting it.

References, Recommended Readings and Resources

1. American Board of Pain Medicine. http://www.abpm.org/what. Accessed July 23, 2018.
2. American Society of Interventional Pain Physicians. http://www.asipp. org/default.html. Last visited July 23, 2018.
3. American Academic Physical Medicine and Rehabilitation. http://www.aapmr.org/education/me. Last visited July 23, 2018.
4. Greg Allen. NPR. The 'Oxy Express': Florida's Drug Abuse Epidemic. March 2, 2011. https://www.npr. org/2011/03/02/134143813/the-oxy-express-floridas-drug-abuse- epidemic. Accessed June 16, 2018.
5. The Oxycontin Express. 2009, DRUGS. https:// topdocumentaryfilms.com/oxycontin-express/. Accessed June 16, 2018.
6. Mariana van Zeller, The Oxycontin Express, Peabody Award-winning edition of Vanguard February 26, 2014. https://www.youtube.com/ watch?v=wGZEvXNqzkM&has_verified=1. Accessed June 16, 2018.
7. Carrie Teegardin. The Atlanta Journal-Constitution. Doctors and the opioid crisis: An AJC National Investigation. December 1, 2017. https://www.myajc.com/news/public-affairs/healers-dealers/ wrKUc6J0p2sz4dFi3fwXJK/. Accessed July 16, 2018.
8. Drug overdose data — https://www.cdc.gov/drugoverdose/data/ statedeaths.html. Accessed June 20, 2018.
9. National Institute on Drug Abuse. Opioid overdose crisis. https:// www.drugabuse.gov/drugs-abuse/opioids/opioid-overdose-crisis. Accessed June 4, 2018.
10 Alana M. Vivolo-Kantor, Ph.D.; Puja Seth, Ph.D.; R. Matthew Gladden,Ph.D.; Christine L. Mattson, Ph.D.; Grant T. Baldwin, Ph.D.; Aaron Kite-Powell, MS; Michael A. Coletta, MPH Vital Signs: Trends in Emergency Department Visits for Suspected Opioid Overdoses — United States, July 2016–September 2017 *March 6, 2018,* MMWR. https://www.cdc.gov/mmwr/volumes/67/wr/mm6709e1.htm. Accessed June 17, 2018.
11. Centers for Disease Control and Prevention. Understanding the Epidemic. https://www.cdc.gov/drugoverdose/epidemic/index.html. Last visited June 16, 2018.
12. Deborah Dowell, MD; Tamara M. Haegerich, Ph.D.; Roger Chou, MD. CDC Guideline for Prescribing Opioids for Chronic Pain. Morbidity and Mortality Weekly Report (MMWR). March 18, 2016. https://www.cdc.gov/mmwr/volumes/65/rr/rr6501e1.htm. Accessed July 23, 2018.
13. Centers for Disease Control and Prevention. CDC prescribing guidelines of 2016. https://www.cdc.gov/drugoverdose/prescribing/ guideline.html. Accessed July 23, 2018.

14. Gery P. Guy Jr., Ph.D.; Kun Zhang, Ph.D.; Michele K. Bohm, MPH; Jan Losby, Ph.D.; Brian Lewis; Randall Young, MA; Louise B. Murphy, Ph.D.; Deborah Dowell, MD· CDCMMWR. Vital Signs: Changes in Opioid Prescribing in the United States, 2006–2015. July 7, 2017 / 66(26);697-704. https://www.cdc.gov/mmwr/volumes/66/wr/mm6626a4.htm?s_cid=mm6626a4_w. Accessed March 1, 2018.

15. Levy B, Paulozzi L, Mack KA, Jones CM. Trends in Opioid Analgesic-Prescribing Rates by Specialty, U.S., 2007-2012. Am J Prev Med. 2015 Sep;49(3):409-13. Apr 18, 2015. Opioid Overdose Prescribing Data - https://www.cdc.gov/drugoverdose/data/prescribing.html. Accessed May 26, 2018.

16. Centers for Disease Control and Prevention. CDC, Opioid Overdose prescribing data https://www.cdc.gov/drugoverdose/data/prescribing. html. Accessed June 10, 2018.

17. Puja Seth, Ph.D.; Lawrence Scholl, Ph.D.; Rose A. Rudd, MSPH; Sarah Bacon, Ph.D., *MMMWR*. Overdose deaths involving opioids, cocaine, and psychostimulants – United States, 2015 – 2016. Centers for Disease Control and Prevention, https://www.cdc.gov/mmwr/ volumes/67/wr/mm6712a1.htm. Accessed May 5, 2018.

18. NIH. National Institute of Drug Abuse. Overdose Death Rates. Revised August 2018. https://www.drugabuse.gov/related-topics/ trends-statistics/overdose-death-rates. Accessed August 16, 2018.

Chapter 3

The other Sixty Percent (60%): Users of Illegal Opioids such as Illicitly Manufactured Fentanyl (IMF), its Synthetic Analogs, Heroin, and others

Sixty percent of all fatal opioid overdoses are directly related to illegal opioids such as heroin and IMF, which is about 50 times as strong as heroin. The other 40% is primarily related to prescription-drug overdoses. These two classes represent 66% of all drug overdoses in the United States, according to the CDC.[1] The use of illegal drugs such as heroin has been around for many years.

There was a heroin epidemic in the 1970s; and in the year 2000, the users' main demographic was primarily minorities aged 45 to 63. The demographics changed by 2013. Now it is primarily young white people aged 18 to 44 that are most affected. However, this is a dynamic process, it continues to affect everyone, and it will not be discriminatory. During the early 1970s and beyond, the primary focus in dealing with drug issues was on law enforcement, resulting in a significant number of incarcerations.

The focus is now trending towards a treatment centered approach, in which the users or opioid addicts are now considered to have a medical problem. IMF was not a major concern at that time compared to heroin.[4]

According to SAMHSA, the number of heroin users increased by 82% from 2007 to 2013 (from 373,00 to 681,000). The CDC also reported that the number of people who fatally overdosed from IMF more than doubled between 2015 and 2016: from 9,580 in 2015 to 19,413 in 2016. During the same time frame, heroin deaths have increased by nearly 20%, whereas the deaths from legally prescribed opioids were up by about 11 %.[2]

Opioids are effective in managing pain and increasing pleasure (although this is not the intention of legally prescribing opioids) by causing dopamine levels to increase. Opioids are very addictive; heroin is one of the most addictive illegal opioids.

It is also believed to have a negative effect by decreasing the user's frontal lobe activities. These brain activities are partly responsible for executive functions such as planning, reasoning, and understanding consequences. In addition, it has a depressing effect on the area of the brain responsible for breathing and respiration. Fentanyl and other legal or illegal opioids have similar effects. The common belief is that users will start out with either illegally or legally prescribed opioids, and subsequently transition to illicit opioids when they are unable to obtain or afford legal prescriptions. With the ever-increasing supplies of illegal drugs, the prices of heroin and IMF have significantly decreased over time, and are now very cheap.

Complicating the issues with illegal opioids is the use of other illegal drugs such as cocaine and marijuana. There are also legally prescribed non-opioid drugs such as benzodiazepines, which includes medication like Xanax and Valium, adding to the problems. The consumption of alcohol also exacerbates the opioid epidemic. The CDC stated that nearly all people who use heroin also use at least one other illegal drug. Also, people who are addicted to alcohol are two times likely, marijuana three times likely, cocaine 15 times likely, and opioids four times more likely to be addicted to heroin. It is reasonable to assume that there are similar correlations with other opioids.[4]

In understanding where we are and calculating from CDC data: of the drug- overdose deaths in the country, legally prescribed opioids represent about 26%, illegal opioids such as heroin and IMF account for about 40%, and non-opioid- related drug overdoses makeup about 34%. All these numbers are significant, and none of these categories stands on its own. Each one has multiple contributing causes that are overlapping. There is no single solution to this overwhelming problem. A meaningful and lasting resolution of this problem is likely only when there is a careful analysis of each of category, with the primary objective of finding comprehensive solutions.

Illegal drugs are a major factor in the opioid epidemic. A significant number of users who become addicted to opioids have never been to a medical doctor or other healthcare providers to manage their addictions or other related problems.[5] They often have no sense of direction, and very little social support related to their drug use and/or addictions.

It is clear that opioid prescriptions had peaked in 2010 and continued to decrease through to 2016. The opioid-death reduction has not paralleled the decline in opioid prescriptions.[6] Despite that, things are heading in the right direction with increased legislation, and greater public and physician/provider awareness.

In addition, changes in the amount and the way opioids are manufactured, distributed and prescribed have affected the availability of legal opioids.

It is now also easier for law enforcement to show up at the offices of medical providers believed to have broken the law, shut them down, and take them to jail. The most significant resistance that may be faced from providers are threats to get their lawyers. The same is not true of illegal drug dealers, even if you think you know where they are. Although efforts have been made to reduce the amount of opioids available to users from illicit dealers, there still remain significant challenges to overcome.

Illegal opioids are still the most significant contributors to opioid-overdose deaths at about 60%. The questions of how illegal drugs are imported by land, sea or air; how much of them are made in this country; where are the drugs coming from; and who are the suppliers, dealers and distributors are questions beyond the scope of this book.

Special Category – Illicitly Manufactured Fentanyl (IMF)

…………ILLICITLY MANUFACTURED FENTANYL (IMF) AND ITS ANALOGS COLLECTIVELY IS THE MOST SIGNIFICANT COMPONENT THREAT OF THE OPIOID EPIDEMIC FACED BY OUR NATION. IT HAS RESULTED IN INCREASINGLY MORE OPIOID RELATED OVERDOSE DEATHS IN UNPRECEDENTED NUMBERS AT A FASTER RATES THAN OTHER OPIOIDS OR ILLEGAL DRUGS PARTICULARLY WITIIIN THE PERIOD OF YEARS 2015 TO 2017. THESE OPIOID OVERDOSE DEATH RATES ARE AMONG THE FASTEST EVER RECORDED AT ANY TIME. THERE IS NO CLEAR OBJECTIVE EVIDENCE OR DATA CURRENTLY AVAILABLE TIIAT WOULD LEAD ONE TO REASONABLE BELIEVE THAT 2018 OR 2019 WILL BE ANY DIFFERENT.

The most significant driving factor in the increase of opioid overdoses is IMF. As indicated above, IMF deaths doubled from 2015 to 2016, whereas heroin increased by 20%, and prescription drugs, by 11%. IMF is very potent: about 50 times more potent than heroin, and about 100 times more potent than morphine. There are also analogs of fentanyl such as carfentanil (and others), which are about 100 times more potent than IMF.[5] The projected data for 2017 shown on the next page is, even more striking with respect to IMF.[18]

Drugs Involved in U.S. Overdose Deaths - *Among the more than 72,000 drug- overdose deaths estimated in 2017, the sharpest increase occurred among deaths related to fentanyl and fentanyl analogs (synthetic opioids), with nearly 30,000 overdose deaths. Source: CDC WONDER. Provisional counts for 2017 are based on data available through 12/17, but are not yet finalized. Counts through 2016 are based on final annual data (more than 20,000 deaths).*

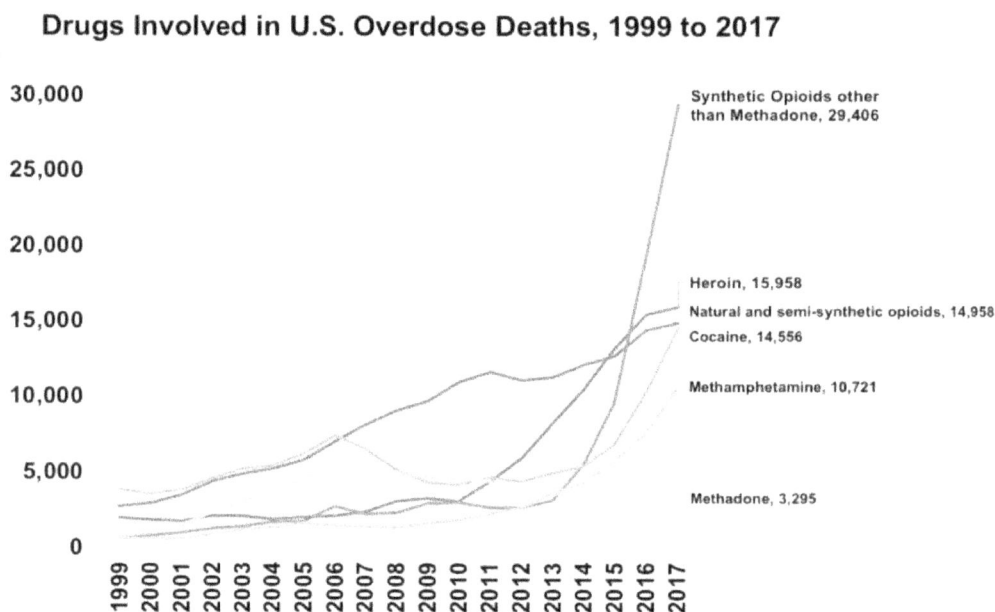

Drugs Involved in U.S. Overdose Deaths, 1999 to 2017

In the figure above, if you look at the synthetic opioids (these include IMF, carfentanil, and others) line, you will notice that it is directly moving up in almost a straight line.

Notice the following from the graph above, between 2002 and 2017:

- overdose deaths from **all opioid drugs** increased more than **four times**
- overdose deaths from **heroin** increased by more than **seven times**
- overdose deaths from **cocaine** increased more than **three times**
- overdose deaths from **methamphetamine** increased more than **five times**
- overdose deaths from illegal **synthetic opioids** such as IMF increased by about **22 times**, doubling between the years 2015 and 2016.

*Not shown in this graph is **benzodiazepines (benzos)** overdose deaths, which increased by more than **eight times** during that period as well.*[17,18]

The Cocaine-and-Opioids Combination Including Synthetic Analog, IMF

You will probably have noticed that all the drugs listed above included legally prescribed opioids and that the overdose deaths from 2002 to 2017 for cocaine alone has increased by more than three times. While its increase is significant, this drug by itself may be considered the least problematic.

However, that is so far from the truth. Cocaine in combination with almost any other legal or illegal drugs can often have devastating consequences. You'll notice in the chart below the increase in deaths by 23 times between the years 2012 and 2016 when cocaine is added to opioids (particularly IMF and other fentanyl analogs).

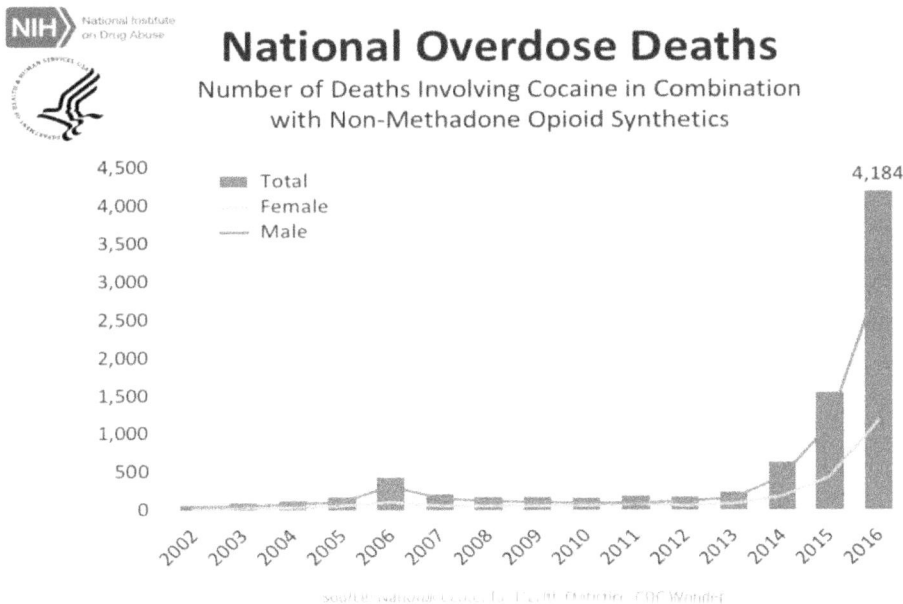

National Overdose Deaths
Number of Deaths Involving Cocaine in Combination
with Non-Methadone Opioid Synthetics

4,184

National Overdose Deaths—Number of Deaths Involving Cocaine in Combination with Non-Methadone Opioid Synthetics. *The figure above is a bar chart showing the total number of U.S. overdose deaths involving cocaine in combination with other synthetic opioids, dominated by IMF. From 2002 to 2016, there was little increase in overall deaths, but from 2012 through 2016, there was a 23-fold increase in the total number of deaths. The chart is overlaid by a line graph showing the number of deaths of females (bottom line) and males (top line) from 2002 to 2016.*[18]

How Potent and Deadly are IMF and the
Other Fentanyl Analogs?

According to the DEA website, as little as 2 mg of IMF (equivalent to the quantity of a few grains of table salt) is enough to cause an overdose, and death in 95% of the American population, if the drugs are ingested.[7] Picture this: if drug dealers/ traffickers of IMF obtain one pound (1 lb) of it, they could then take that one pound and divide that into about 450 equal portions. They could then take each portion and divide them into 1000 portions each of 1 mg.

Therefore, these dealers/traffickers could potentially make about 450,000 pills with 1 mg of IMF in each, or 225,000 pills with 2 mg of IMF in each. If they decide to use 2 mg, each pill may be fatal to the non-opioid-using or opioid-naïve individuals. Fortunately, they're not the ones being sold these pills most of the time. For their customers, they may settle somewhere between 1 mg and 3 mg, which may or may not be fatal depending on who is consuming or ingesting it.

What else goes into the making of each pill as filler is entirely up to the dealers/traffickers. Fillers are other compounds added to make fake pills and may include other opioids or other illegal drugs like cocaine, methamphetamine, or heroin. The emergence of fake pills laced with illicit drugs such as IMF, and worse, carfentanil (remember, that's 100 times more potent than IMF!) continues to rise as a source of diversion, and other legal supplies become harder to obtain. The fake pills are sometimes sold as Percocet, oxycodone or hydrocodone (among other legally prescribed opioids), and at much lower prices than authentic medications.

This is an excellent business for dealers and traffickers because they could sell each pill anywhere from about $10-$20; their initial expense for one pound of IMF may cost them a few thousand dollars, but they could potentially net millions. This is scary on so many levels, to say the least.[8]

If you still have not figured out how scary and crazy this is, let me add one other thought. The DEA seized 12 kg of IMF in Northeast California, and 40 kg in Atlanta, Georgia during a traffic stop back in May 2016. The total haul was 52 kg of IMF.[8] This amount of IMF could make more than 20 million to 25 million 2-mg pills, enough to kill that many people.

So, do not get too excited when you see your favorite "pain doctors" on the evening news, heading off to jail. This although probably justify, is often the symptoms of a much larger problem. As I have indicated, discussing or addressing issues related to drug trafficking or the importation or manufacture of illegal drugs is beyond the scope of this book.

Designer or Synthetic/Analog Drugs of Opioids and Others

The demand for more opioids increases as the supplies of the usual channels are either cut off, or the amount usually available from them is greatly reduced for any number of reasons. This has led to a class of drugs referred to as designer or synthetic/analog drugs. Some of these designer drugs' manufacturers have as their primary goal the production of opioid-like drugs. Analog drugs result from slight modifications of known drugs, with the new compound having properties similar to the old one. This can result in compounds that are very similar to or very different from the original opioids.

Sometimes, the new synthetic drugs are more potent than the original one, or it may be less effective than the one it is modeled after. For example, carfentanil, which is an IMF analog, is about 100 times more potent than IMF. In turn, IMF is about 50 times as potent as heroin. In other words, carfentanil is about 5000 times as potent as heroin. By creating analogs, the new drugs may have routes of ingestion that were unavailable for the parent compounds. Also, the mechanism of action, or the way the drugs function to produce their effects may be markedly different.

Resulting from this are different opioids and other compounds with varying effects and can cause catastrophic consequences. In addition, the way most opioid-overdose patients are treated with conventional medication such as naloxone/Narcan may not be as effective. In some cases, if it is effective, it may require larger doses than what is expected for a typical opioid overdose.

Opioid users also may mix other opioids or illegal drugs such as cocaine with one of the main drugs they are taking, essentially creating a drug cocktail. This is extremely dangerous, and can often be fatal. There is also the addition of various types of compounds or substances that the dealers, suppliers or distributors often add before it gets to the actual users to maximize profits. Here, there is zero consideration for safety or any resulting adverse consequence.

The users are always at the highest risk for catastrophic things happening to them because, in almost all instances, they are incapable or unable to determine the purity of the drugs that they are taking. Often, they have no idea if their current new stock of drugs will create their last high.

Also, the suppliers who are selling or giving the users the drugs may very often have no idea what is contained in the drugs they are selling or giving away. They may be just as ignorant as the users. Their job is to sell or distribute the products given to them and in the process make money.

It is conceivable therefore that they will have no or very little reason to feel guilty about the consequence of the users being affected adversely by their action, after all, all they did was provide the drugs; the users have the option of refusing to take it.

Legal fentanyl prescribed for individual patients is administered by a transdermal patch (through the skin) or an injection into the muscle or intravenously. The IMF is usually in pill or powder form; it can then be made into a liquid or a solution which allows for it to be consumed by injection, snorting or swallowing. Because of its potency, there is usually a substantial amount of additives/substances that increase the amounts and profitability of these drugs. Fentanyl's overdose deaths numbers show that IMF and its analogs are much deadlier than traditional opioids. Analog of fentanyl such as such as carfentanil, although not generally as readily available as IMF, is becoming more accessible, and it can be fatal by just skin contact. It is believed to be about 100 times more potent than IMF.

Many of these analog drugs can be sold cheaply, thus making the opioid epidemic much worse. Not only are they sold in person, but they are also sold online, often being disguised in part by labeling such as "not approved for human or animal consumption." Some designer drugs may even be sold over- the-counter at convenient stores or gas stations long before the dangers are realized, and significant damage has already been done. The naming and marketing of these drugs allow them to appear harmless or benign to most consumers. There are numerous synthetic drugs; some are more well-known than others.

Flakka: Synthetic Cathianone. This is a designer drug that has resulted in significant harm to many of its users. It is also called gravel, bath salts or alpha- PVP, among others. It is extremely addictive, and its use is associated with psychosis and paranoia. Its effect is sometimes compared to that of cocaine.

However, it is much more potent and cheaper. Its use has also been reported to cause "excited delirium" signs and symptoms ranging from elevated temperature, kidney failure, hallucination, and increased strength. The user may also become depressed and/or suicidal with increased violent tendencies.[9,10,14]

Designer drug U-47700, also called Pink, was sold on the internet, and frequently used or mixed with other drugs such as heroin and or IMF. This resulted in several fatal overdoses. This drug was subsequently banned by the DEA and classified as Schedule I.[13,14]

Synthetic forms of cannabinoids. Although they are non-opioids, variants like Spice or K2 are believed to have similar properties to THC, and generally considered more dangerous concerning its potential adverse effects.[15]

Some of these designer drugs are regional and short-lived, and many have been born out of either an attempt to make the parent drugs or create new compounds believed to result in a greater high. Sometimes, the result is just a mixture that will vary according to what is added and how much, without any specific new compound being generated or synthesized. In June 2017, a so-called manufactured "Percocet" was sold in Central and South Georgia (in the Macon and Perry areas), resulting in several hospitalizations and fatal overdoses.[11,12,15]

Another combination drug that is often deadly and found its way in the hands of the unsuspecting opioid users often resulting in overdose deaths is a mixed compound called **Gray Death.** This may be composed of a mixture of heroin, fentanyl, carfentanil, U – 47700 and possibly other synthetic opioids. There is no specific known proportion in which these drugs are added together or which ones are included. One thing for sure is that each of these drugs alone can kill anyone. Therefore, it shouldn't be a surprise that combining them together to create a more potent compound or create a greater high will definitely in most cases lead to deadly consequences. Sometimes, just by virtue of physical contact with Gray Death may lead to drug overdose and possible deaths particularly in cases of opioid naïve individuals.[15]

The Federal Analog Act, 21 U.S.C. § 813 of 1986

Considering the overwhelming number of designer drugs and attempts to make more of them, **the Federal Analog Act, 21 U.S.C. § 813** was passed in 1986, making it illegal to manufacture designer analog compounds that are similar to illicit drugs.[15] This means that, for example, if someone is trying to manufacture an illegal drug that's similar in structure, properties or function to a known Schedule I drug, the new drug (although unknown to the federal government/DEA) will also be an illegal Schedule I drug. Therefore, the same laws would apply as for the known drugs because the new one was manufactured to be comparable to it.

References, Recommended Readings and Resources

1. Centers for Disease Control and Prevention. That Understanding the Epidemic. https://www.cdc.gov/drugoverdose/epidemic/index.html. Last visited June 16, 2018.
2. U.S. drug overdose deaths continue to rise; increase fueled by synthetic opioids. https://www.cdc.gov/media/releases/2018/p0329- drug-overdose-deaths.html. Accessed May 5, 2018.
3. Overdose deaths involving opioids, cocaine, and psychostimulants – the United States, 2015 – 2016. https://www.cdc.gov/mmwr/ volumes/67/wr/mm6712a1.htm. Accessed May 5, 2018.
4. Centers for Disease Control and Prevention. Today's Heroin Epidemic https://www.cdc.gov/vitalsigns/heroin/index.html. Accessed April 10, 2018.
5. Puja Seth, Ph.D.; Lawrence Scholl, Ph.D.; Rose A. Rudd, MSPH; Sarah Bacon, Ph.D., *MMMWR*. Overdose deaths involving opioids, cocaine, and psychostimulants – United States, 2015 – 2016. https:// www.cdc.gov/mmwr/volumes/67/wr/mm6712a1.htm. Accessed May 5, 2018.
6. Gery P. Guy Jr., Ph.D.; Kun Zhang, Ph.D.; Michele K. Bohm, MPH; Jan Losby, Ph.D.; Brian Lewis; Randall Young, MA; Louise B. Murphy, Ph.D.; Deborah Dowell, MD. CDCMMWR. Vital Signs: Changes in Opioid Prescribing in the United States, 2006–2015. July 7, 2017 / 66(26);697-704.
7. Centers for Disease Control and Prevention. https://www.cdc. gov/mmwr/volumes/66/wr/mm6626a4.htm?s_cid=mm6626a4_w. Accessed March 1, 2018.
8. Drug Enforcement Administration. FAQ's-Fentanyl and Fentanyl- Related Substances. https://www.dea.gov/druginfo/fentanyl-faq.shtml. Accessed June 1, 2018.
9. Centers for Disease Control and Prevention. Opioid Overdose Prescribing Data- https://www.cdc.gov/drugoverdose/data/prescribing. html. Accessed May 26, 2018.
10. Penders TM, Gestring RE, Vilensky DA. Excited delirium following the use of synthetic cathinones (bath salts). Gen Hosp Psychiatry. 2012 Nov-Dec;34(6):647-50. https://www.ncbi.nlm.nih.gov/ pubmed/22898445. Last visited April 2, 2018.
11. National Institute on Drug Abuse. Commonly Abused Drugs Charts. https://www.drugabuse.gov/drugs-abuse/commonly-abused-drugs- charts. Accessed April 2, 2018.
12. Rhonda Cook. AJC.COM. Death toll rises in mass overdose in Middle Georgia. June 06, 2017. https://www.ajc.com/news/ crime--law/death-toll-rises-mass-overdose-middle-georgia/pH6cM5ifTL95wCDGJ9c3lK/?icmp=np_inform_variation-control. Accessed July 24, 2018.
13. Corky Siemaszko. NBCNews.com. Opioid Crisis Batters Georgia as Suspicious Percocet Kills Two. Jun.06.2017. https://www.nbcnews. com/storyline/americas-heroin-epidemic/opioid-crisis-batters-georgia- suspicious-percocet-kills-two-n768951. Accessed July 24, 2018.

14. Tracy Connor. NBC News.com. Feds Move to Ban Pink, Heroin Substitute That's Killed Dozens. Nov.10.2016. https://www.nbcnews. com/news/us-news/feds-move-ban-pink-heroin-substitute-s-killed- dozens-n682106. Accessed July 24, 2018.

15. NIH. Emerging Trends and Alerts | National Institute on Drug Abuse (NIDA). https://www.drugabuse.gov/drugs-abuse/emerging-trends- alerts. Accessed July 24, 2018.

16. Drug Enforcement Administration. Diversion Control Division. Title 21 United States Code (USC) Controlled Substances Act. Oct. 27, 1986. https://www.deadiversion.usdoj.gov/21cfr/21usc/813.htm. Accessed July 24, 2018.

17. Benzodiazepines and Opioids | National Institute on Drug Abuse (NIDA). March 2018. https://www.drugabuse.gov/drugs-abuse/ opioids/benzodiazepines-opioids. Accessed June 10, 2018.

18. NIH. National Institute of Drug Abuse. Overdose Death Rates. Revised August 2018. https://www.drugabuse.gov/related-topics/ trends-statistics/overdose-death-rates. Accessed August 16, 2018.

Chapter 4

The Other Thirty-four (34%) of Non-Opioids: Users of Cocaine, Methamphetamine, Benzodiazepines, and Others

There are three main classes of drug overdoses in the United States. The first one is related to prescriptions of **legal opioids**. The second is caused by **illegal opioids** such as IMF and heroin. These two together account for about 66% of total drug overdoses in 2016 according to the CDC and are primarily responsible for the opioid epidemic. The other 34% are caused by **non-opioids such as legal prescription drugs** like central nervous system depressants, benzodiazepines, sleep aids or even alcohol.

In addition, there are also **non-opioid illegal drugs** including central nervous system depressants and stimulants, hallucinogens or psychoactive substances that contributed to a significant number of deaths. Some of these are cocaine, methamphetamine, designer drugs, LSD, PCP, and ecstasy-MDMA. Deaths from drug overdoses often range from a single drug to multiple drugs of different combinations, some of which may be legal and others, illegal. A total of over 63,600 people in the United States died of drug overdoses in 2016, and more than 21,000 people died from non-opioid-related drug overdoses.[1,2] It is now estimated that in the year 2017 more than 72,000 people have died from all drug overdose [10]

The Benzo Express – Heading to a Town Near You and Your Favorite Place

Benzodiazepines (benzos) are essentially a group of legally prescribed sedatives for the treatment of anxiety, sleep disorder/insomnia, and muscle spasms, among others. Common examples are alprazolam (Xanax), diazepam (Valium), lorazepam (Ativan), and clonazepam (Klonopin).

They have the effect of calming or sedating patients. However, because they are central nervous system depressants, they also have adverse effects on the respiratory/breathing center of the brain, similar to opioids and alcohol. Therefore, they significantly increase the risk of death when taken with either opioids, alcohol, or both.[3]

Benzos also carry with them significant risks of tolerance and dependence- associated withdrawals and addiction similar to opioids. However, this is often not emphasized or discussed with patients when they are prescribed these medications, sometimes resulting in them not being fully aware of the dangers of taking them.

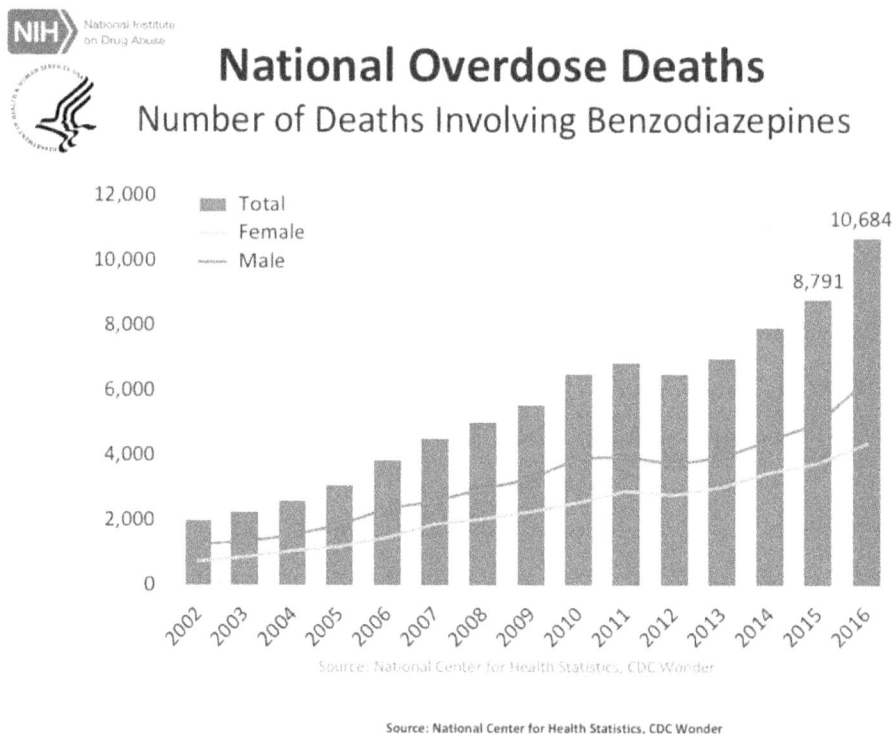

National Overdose Deaths
Number of Deaths Involving Benzodiazepines

Source: National Center for Health Statistics, CDC Wonder

National Overdose Deaths—Number of Deaths Involving Benzodiazepines *The figure above is a bar chart showing the total number of U.S. overdose deaths involving benzodiazepines from 2002 to 2016. The chart is overlaid by a line graph showing the number of deaths of females (bottom line) and males (top line).* **From 2002 to 2016, there was an eightfold increase in the total number of deaths.**[10]

While most medications are tested and approved for use, there are dangers and side effects that are sometimes fatal, particularly when the medications are not used as intended to or as prescribed.

In 2002, less than 2,000 people died from overdoses related to benzos. In 2015, this number went up to around 9,000. These numbers represent a quadrupling of deaths associated with benzos, and almost parallels the rising deaths of the opioid epidemic over a similar period.[8,10] But these numbers are changing very quickly. Between 2002 and 2016, there was an eightfold increase in the total number of deaths involving benzos, as shown in the next graph (next page). This resulted because of the significant increase in the number of overdose deaths that occurred in 2016

The Similarities of Benzos and Opioids in the Era of the Opioid Epidemic

One of the most vibrant phases of the opioid epidemic occurred in Florida in the late 1990s and went on until around 2010. This was a time when opioids, specifically OxyContin and other opioids and controlled substances, were prescribed in Florida by physicians/providers in quantities that were greater in total than all other states combined. Since then, Florida has enacted the so-called Pill mill Laws and other regulations as well as implementing the state Prescription Drugs Monitoring Program (PDMP). These have virtually eliminated or drastically reduced Pill mills and doctor-shopping, essentially restoring Florida to a state which no longer has the largest number of opioid prescribers. But it has also seen a significant reduction in the number of prescriptions written by their providers, and its numbers now fall within the range of other states.[4,5]

In 2017, the Medical Examiners Commission of Florida's Department of Law Enforcement issued its annual report of 2016 on Drugs Identified in Deceased Persons for that year. Opioids, both from legal prescriptions and illegal drugs, still remained a significant cause of fatal overdoses.

However, deaths (1,421) from benzos such as alprazolam (Xanax), diazepam (Valium) and others have now surpassed those (723) from OxyContin/oxycodone, which was once a significant cause of deaths in that state.[6,7] Florida is by no means alone in the rise of benzos as the cause of deaths in their states.

Across the country and in just about every state, the prescriptions and use of benzos are out of control. Sadly, this is significantly reflected by the increase in overdoses and deaths of patients or individuals who use both opioids and benzos. According to the CDC, more than 30% of overdoses involving opioids also involve benzos.[8]

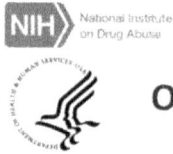

Opioid Involvement in Benzodiazepine Overdose

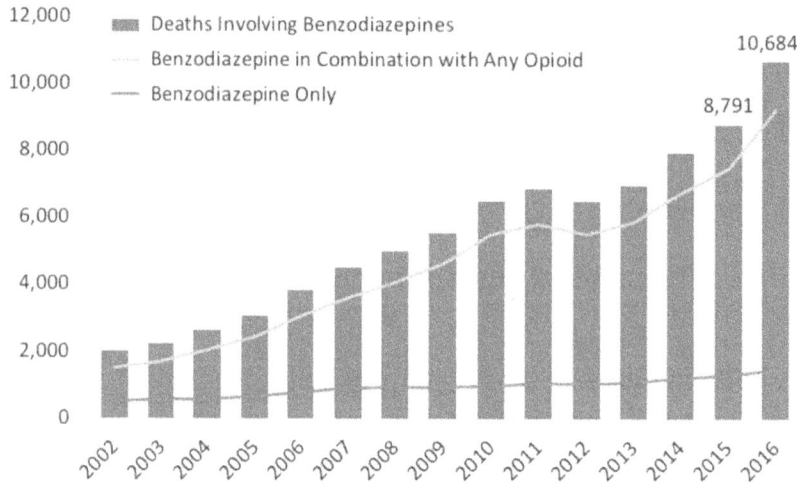

Source: National Center for Health Statistics, CDC Wonder

National Overdose Deaths—Number of Deaths Involving Benzodiazepines, with and without opioids. *Benzodiazepines from 2002 to 2016, with the yellow line (top) representing the number of benzodiazepine deaths that also involved opioids, and the orange line (bottom) representing benzodiazepine deaths that did not involve opioids. From 2002-2016, benzodiazepine deaths involving opioids increased six-fold, more than those not involving opioids.[10,10]*

So, Why Is This?

Do you realize that by far, most benzo prescriptions are written with refills? These refills range from three months, six months or one year. This simply means that once most patients see their doctors for evaluation/face-to-face monitoring, they don't have to see them again for another three months to one year. If you are a patient or pharmacists filling these prescriptions, you will notice that these prescriptions invariably have multiple refills. The next question that is often asked is: who are the doctors/providers writing these prescriptions? In a similar manner to pain management, the answer would be primary care, internal medicine/family practitioners, and mid-levels, and then psychiatrists and associates who work in mental health services who have specific expertise in managing patients who need these medications.

The challenges have always been, however, that there is not enough psychiatrists or related specialists/providers who can address the demands of the number of patients/individuals using these medications. Therefore, the task of writing these medications goes to primary care providers and associates. But what is most troubling is that the risks for diversions, misuse and abuse are far more significant than that of opioids.

Part of the reason for this is a gross lack of awareness of benzos and its impact on society as a whole and the opioid epidemic in particular. Added to this is the minimal monitoring of their use by the patients who receive these medications, often in substantial quantities. Most providers have limited objective ways of monitoring the prescriptions they give to their patients.

In fact, the few times some patients are truly monitored are when they present to pain management clinics, which monitor them as part of their standard of care. Many of us in pain management service can attest to the fact that very often, we will ask these patients when they last took their benzos. The typical responses are "as needed" and, in some common scenarios several months ago, "because I'm doing better now." However, when you look at their state's PDMP, they or others related to them have **not** failed in picking up their prescriptions like clockwork every month. What is sometimes also shocking is the providers' responses when you call their offices or send them a correspondence indicating that their patients are not taking their prescribed medications.

They are often at a loss for words or simply do nothing. This allows us to believe that if a patient is diverging, misusing and/or abusing other prescribers' medications, that patient is also likely to be doing the same with the ones we prescribed. Therefore, any patient found to be displaying these behaviors should be considered to have acceptable reasons for discharge from pain management practice if corrective measures cannot be implemented.

There are similar situations with medications such as Addcrall and antidepressants. Alcohol, which is entirely legal, is often taken for granted and is used in abundance with benzos, opioids, or a combination of the three.

These medications also need to be monitored, of course. As providers, we keep emphasizing the need to avoid at all costs mixing benzos and opioids, as well the need to avoid alcohol with either of these. In addition, you should never combine all three, because the rates of overdose and death are significantly increased.

What about Cocaine and Other Drugs?

Although cocaine and many other psychostimulants, hallucinogens or central nervous system stimulants are not opioids, they still play a significant role in the opioid epidemic (see tables in the Appendix for commonly used psychostimulants, hallucinogens, and opioids; as well as some of their street names).

Any number of these substances may be found at any time from conducted autopsies related to drug overdoses. Sometimes, they are present without opioids; other times, opioids are present; although they may not be significant in the cause of death. However, like benzos and other substances, they form a considerable portion of drugs responsible for overdoses that at times may be relevant in the presence of the opioid epidemic. The CDC analysts, based on 2015 to 2016 data, revealed that cocaine-related overdose deaths increased by 52.4% and psychostimulant-related overdose deaths increased by 33.3%. These are compared with the heroin-related death rate that increased by 19.5%, prescription-related overdose deaths increased by 10.6%, and alarmingly, synthetic opioids probably related to IMF increased by more than 100% (the overdose rates more than doubled).

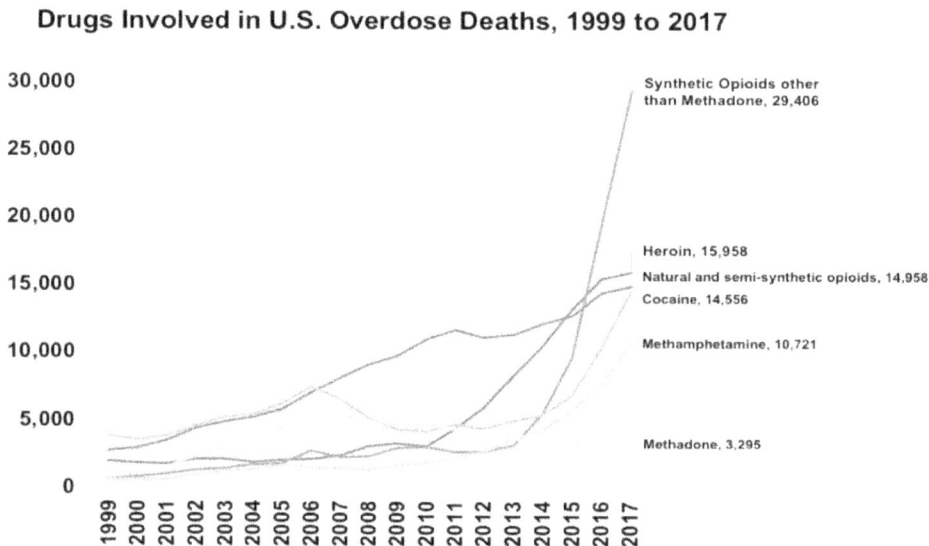

Drugs Involved in U.S. Overdose Deaths, 1999 to 2017

Synthetic Opioids other than Methadone, 29,406
Heroin, 15,958
Natural and semi-synthetic opioids, 14,958
Cocaine, 14,556
Methamphetamine, 10,721
Methadone, 3,295

Drugs Involved in U.S. Overdose Deaths - *Among the more than 72,000 drug- overdose deaths estimated in 2017, the sharpest increase occurred among deaths related to fentanyl and fentanyl analogs (synthetic opioids), with nearly 30,000 overdose deaths. Source: CDC WONDER. Provisional counts for 2017 are based on data available through 12/17, but are not yet finalized. Counts through 2016 are based on final annual data.*[10]

Clearly, both opioids and non-opioids are significantly outpacing the rate of deaths compared to prescription drugs.[2] Moreover, the numbers continue to rise as shown by analyzing the projected data for 2017 deaths.[10] The impact of **cocaine in combination with opioids** was discussed in Chapter 3. The combination showed a **23-fold increase in deaths** when opioids and IMF were combined with cocaine between **2012 and 2016.**[10]

One thing to bear in mind is that although this is an opioid epidemic, the other drugs and/or stimulants/substances that are available and had been available have simply not disappeared. Invariably, multiple drugs/substances are identified in a significant number of individuals who died from an overdose. Sometimes, it is difficult for medical examiners or pathologists to determine which substance is most likely responsible for the deaths of some of those who overdosed.[12]

Another useful thing to remember is the **correlation between non-opioids and opioid-related deaths or overdoses**. A good example of this is heroin, the use of which has been a significant component of illegal drugs in the United States. The CDC reports that all individuals who use heroin use at least one other drug, while most use at least three other drugs. The CDC report further states that people who are addicted to alcohol are two times, marijuana three times, cocaine 15 times, and prescription painkillers 40 times more likely to be addicted to heroin.[11] Now, if you say to yourself "I don't do heroin," understand that heroin is an opioid and that other opioids have similar or even the same effects like it, sometimes much worse. It is also worth mentioning that youths or individuals who misuse marijuana at an early age are at a much higher risk of misusing opioids than those who do not.

References, Recommended Readings and Resources

1. U.S. drug overdose deaths continue to rise; increase fueled by synthetic opioids. https://www.cdc.gov/media/releases/2018/p0329- drug-overdose-deaths.html. Accessed May 5, 2018.
2. Puja Seth, Ph.D.; Lawrence Scholl, Ph.D.; Rose A. Rudd, MSPH; Sarah Bacon, Ph.D., *MMMWR.* Overdose deaths involving opioids, cocaine, and psychostimulants – the United States, 2015 – 2016. https://www.cdc.gov/mmwr/volumes/67/wr/mm6712a1.htm. Accessed May 5, 2018.
3. National Institute on Drug Abuse. Commonly Abused Drugs Charts. https://www.drugabuse.gov/drugs-abuse/commonly-abused-drugs- charts. Accessed April 2, 2018.
4. Greg Allen -NPR. The 'Oxy Express': Florida's Drug Abuse Epidemic. March 2, 2011. https://www.npr. org/2011/03/02/134143813/the-oxy-express-floridas-drug-abuse- epidemic. Accessed June 16, 2018.
5. The Oxycontin Express. 2009, DRUGS. https://topdocumentaryfilms.com/oxycontin-express. Accessed June 16, 2018.
6. Drugs identified in deceased persons by Florida medical examiners - https://www.fdle.state.fl.us/MEC/Publications-and-Forms/Documents/ Drugs-in-Deceased-Persons/2016-Annual-Drug-Report.aspx. Accessed June 6, 2018.
7. Florida Medical Examiner's Report. http://www.flpdmpfoundation. com/2016/04/28/florida-medical-examiners-report. Accessed June 6, 2018.
8. Benzodiazepines and Opioids | National Institute on Drug Abuse (NIDA). March 2018. https://www.drugabuse.gov/drugs-abuse/ opioids/benzodiazepines-opioids. Accessed June 10, 2018.
9. Centers for Disease Control and Prevention (CDC). National Vital Statistics System, Mortality. CDC WONDER Online Database. https://wonder.cdc.gov/. Published 2017.
10. NIH. National Institute of Drug Abuse. Overdose Death Rates. https:// www.drugabuse.gov/related-topics/trends-statistics/overdose-death- rates. Accessed August 16, 2018.
11. Centers for Disease Control and Prevention. Today's Heroin Epidemic. https://www.cdc.gov/vitalsigns/heroin/index.html. Accessed April 10, 2018.
12. Margaret Warner, Ph.D., James P. Trinidad, M.P.H., M.S., Brigham A. Bastian, B.S., Arialdi M. Miniño, M.P.H., and Holly Hedegaard, M.D., M.S.P.H. Drugs Most Frequently Involved in Drug Overdose Deaths: the United States, 2010–2014 by National Center for Health Statistics. Volume 65 number 10. December 28, 2016. https://www.cdc.gov/ nchs/data/nvsr/nvsr65/nvsr65_10.pdf. Last accessed June 23, 2018.

Chapter 5

The Prescription Diversions of Opioids and Other Controlled Substances

Diversions of prescription medications have always been a factor in our lives, ranging from friends sharing medications to loved ones sharing whatever they have. The sharing of medications is not uncommon, particularly when it comes to medications that those involved believe will cause little or no harm at all. Hence, the prevalence of opioids and other controlled substances' diversion continues to increase. There are a significant number of individuals who falsely believe that sharing these medications is essentially safe, but nothing could be further from the truth. In addition, there is also the sharing of illegal drugs or substances among individuals or friends or loved ones.

The overprescription of opioids between 1999 and 2010 is believed by many to be the central reason for the current opioid epidemic. During that period, opioid prescriptions quadrupled. Also noted was a corresponding increase in opioid- overdose deaths, which increased from the year 1999 to fivefold in CDC data indicated that legal opioids caused 40% of opioid deaths, and 60% were caused by illegal opioids like heroin and IMF. The total of all deaths from opioid overdose in 2016 was over 42,000.[2] It is projected that more than 49,000 died in 2017.[6]

Of all the opioids prescribed, about 53% were diverted to family, friends, and sometimes directly for sale to customers. Some of these opioids will be used recreationally or sold to patients who are in pain but cannot afford to go to doctors or are unlikely to be accepted in a legitimate pain clinic.[3]

Source Where Pain Relievers Were Obtained for Most Recent Nonmedical Use among Past Year Users Aged 12 or Older: 2012-2013[3]

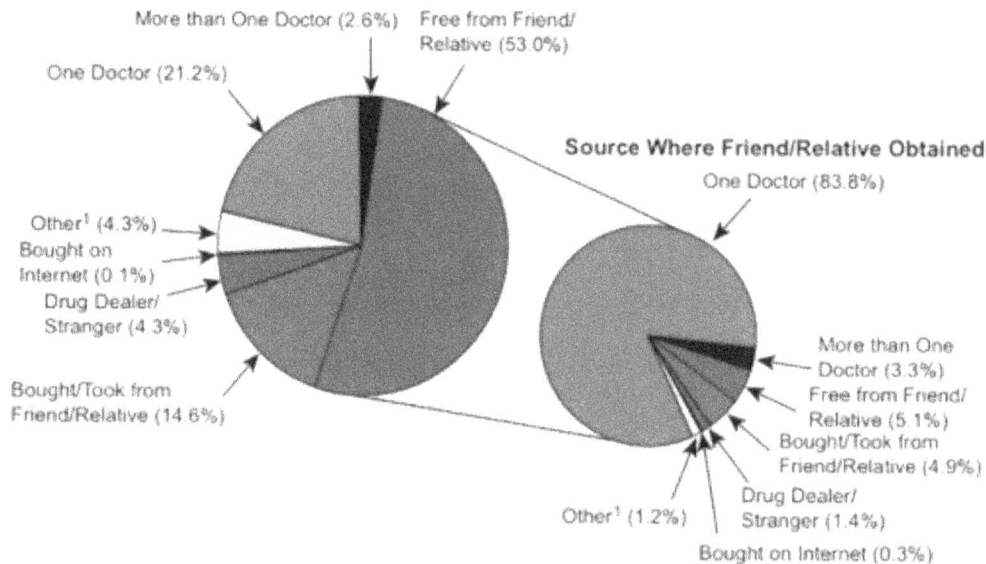

Source Where User Obtained Pain Relievers

[1]*The Other category includes the sources "Wrote Fake Prescription," "Stole from Doctor's Office/Clinic/Hospital/Pharmacy," and "Some Other Way." Note: The percentages do not add to 100 percent due to rounding.*

These customers/patients will continue to use these medications, sometimes for free or at a very high price, until the supplies run out. Once this occurs, the illegal opioids such as heroin and IMF, which are much cheaper and more easily accessible, often fill the void; and continuing the path to drug dependency, possible addiction, and deaths.

The Challenge of Diversions

The challenge of diversions is that there are so many different ways and options that contribute to this significant problem. This may lead to misuse, abuse, addiction, deaths, and a trail of destruction along the path travel.

Diversions may start as simple as giving a friend or family member an opioid pill. From there, things escalate. Very often, older folks present to a pain clinic or their primary care physicians office with complaints of pain and are prescribed significant doses of opioids, most of which they never take, or it is taken away from them by other family members or caregivers.

The elderly are not the only victims. In some cases, there are also strong and healthy people who either directly or indirectly add to the problem of diversions. This is very common when patients are overtreated with large doses of opioids for problems that are minor or problems that could be treated more conservatively or without opioids.

There are many places where diversions occur: hospitals, nursing homes, skilled nursing facilities, pharmacies, personal care homes, and through general health professional/providers who dispense or come in contact with opioids.

The reductions in diversions require a multidimensional approach. All healthcare providers who write prescriptions should carefully assess the needs to continue opioids, and specifically, the amount and/or quantities their patients are receiving. Also, frequent and appropriate monitoring with urine drug screens for use and compliance are extremely essential. Medication review, pill counts and frequent reviews of states' PDMP are also invaluable tools.

In institutions and facilities, cameras and computerized prescription dispensing carts have proven useful. However, they too have limits; one cannot cover all places with a camera, and neither can a computer dispense medication directly to the patients. There's also an expense factor, with so many facilities unable to afford electronic dispensing carts or appropriate cameras in their facilities to help reduce diversions. Hence, we all have to rely on each other and monitor each other as we face the challenges of the opioid epidemic.

Congress passed **The Controlled Substances Act** (CSA) in 1970. The legislation was partly intended to reduce or eliminate diversions by controlling the amount of narcotics available and are prescribed.

Disposal of Opioids and Other Controlled Substances

With respect to the disposal of unused opioids and other controlled substances, the DEA made available for its implementation **The Secure and Responsible Drug Disposal Act of 2010**, also called the Disposal Act. It amended the CSA, giving the DEA the authority to regulate how unused narcotics are disposed of. The primary objective of this was to control diversions.

There are established collection points or sites throughout the country that are registered with the DEA to collect unused controlled substances for destruction. With the opioid epidemic being of major concern, in addition to issues related to the diversions of narcotics, the expectation is that more sites will be registered for collections.

The DEA had designated April 28, 2018, as **National Prescription Drug Take Back Day**. On that day, between 10 AM and 2 PM, centers/sites across the country provided safe and convenient places for collecting unused prescription drugs. Part of the program is also meant to educate the public about the potential for medications abuse, primarily opioids. The first National Prescription Drug Take Back Event was held on September 25, 2010. The campaign was done in all 50 states and collected more than 121 tons of prescription pills. This was considered a great success. It was then followed by subsequent National Prescription Drug Take Back Days that occurred roughly twice per year. The April 28, 2018 event has seen the largest single record collection so far, surpassing that of October 2017.

The total number of law enforcement participation was 4,683, and the total weight of drugs collected was 474.5 tons compared to 456 tons in October 2017. There was also a larger number of sites available for collection on April 28: 5,842 compared to about 5,300 back in October 2017.

Since the inception of the program, more than 4,980 tons of drugs have been collected. The last National Prescription Drug Take Back Day in 2018 was on October 27. [5] The success of this program has grown over the years; it has continued to remove a considerable amount of opioids as well as other controlled substances that have a very high probability of being part of a larger diversions pool. The removal of some unwanted/unused control substances (particularly opioids) from diversions will make some difference in saving lives.

Prior to and after modifications to some of these bills and/or regulations, most of the packages and instructions that come with medications and/or instructions given to patients usually involved the recommendation that patients flush their narcotics down the toilet. This recommendation is disappearing fast.

It is now apparent to most people and providers that a significant number of these medications never got flushed. Therefore, this potentially increases the amount available for diversions, misuse, and abuse.

However, there is still controversy concerning what patients need to do with their unused medications, as a significant number of pharmaceutical inserts still recommend that they be flushed.

The Justice Department and the DEA Proposed Significant Opioids and Other Controlled Substances' Manufacturing Reduction

The federal government, specifically the DEA, determines the number of medications that various pharmaceutical companies produce each year in the United States. It does this in part by examining and analyzing sales data, usage and surplus, among other factors. It proposed what is called an Aggregate Production Quota (APQ) for each class and/or type of medication or compound. The DEA determined in 2017 to set a quota to reduce the production of all Schedule II opioids in the United States by 25% or more. Oxycodone and hydrocodone were specifically set to be reduced to 66% of the 2016 quota. This decision was in part because of the decrease in demand for Schedule II opioids. This would also help control the number of opioids being diverted for illegal use and or abuse. For 2018, a further reduction of about 20% was proposed and is currently in effect for similar reasons. [5,7,8].

SEE THE TABLE OF OPIOID REDUCTION ON THE NEXT PAGE

There were 11.8 million people over the age of 12 years old who misused opioids in 2016. Most of them (11.5 million) were misusing pain relievers rather than heroin.[9]

The Proposal and Reduction since 2016 Shown in the Table below

For the Six Opioids As of August 21, 2018.

Both Aggregate Production Quota for Opioids (grams)	2016	2017		2018		2019 (proposed)		Overall
Fentanyl	2,300,000	1,350,000	41%	1,342,320	1%	1,185,000	12%	-48%
Hydrocodone (for sale)	86,000,000	51,900,000	40%	50,348,280	3%	44,710,000	11%	-48%
Hydromorphone	7,000,000	5,140,800	27%	4,547,720	12%	4,071,000	10%	-42%
Morphine (for sale)	62,500,000	35,000,000	44%	33,958,440	3%	31,450,000	7%	-50%
Oxycodone (for sale)	139,150,000	101,500,000	27%	95,692,000	6%	85,578,000	11%	-38%
Oxymorphone (for sale)	6,250,000	3,600,000	42%	3,395,280	6%	2,880,000	5%	-54%
Overall Decline:	303,200,000	198,490,800	35%	189,284,040	5%	169,874,000	10%	-44%

References, Recommended Readings and Resources

1. Gery P. Guy Jr., Ph.D.; Kun Zhang, Ph.D.; Michele K. Bohm, MPH; Jan Losby, Ph.D.; Brian Lewis; Randall Young, MA; Louise B. Murphy, Ph.D.; Deborah Dowell, MD· CDCMMWR Vital Signs: Changes in Opioid Pre- scribing in the United States, 2006–2015. July 7, 2017, / 66(26);697–704. https://www.cdc.gov/mmwr/volumes/66/ wr/mm6626a4.htm?s_cid=m- m6626a4_w. Accessed March 1, 2018.

2. Center for Disease Control and Prevention. Understanding the Epidemic. https://www.cdc.gov/drugoverdose/epidemic/index.html. Last visited June 16, 2018.

3. SAMHSA. Results from the 2013 National Survey on Drug Use and Health: Summary of National Findings. https://www.samhsa. gov/data/sites/de- fault/files/NSDUHresultsPDFWHTML2013/Web/ NSDUHresults2013. htm. Last visited July 12, 2018.

4. Justice Department, DEA Propose Significant Opioid Manufacturing Re- duction in 2019. August 16, 2018.https://www.justice.gov/opa/pr/ jus- tice-department-dea-propose-significant-opioid-manufacturing-reduction-2019. Last visited August 21, 2018.

5. Drug Enforcement Administration: Diversion Control Division. National Prescription Drug Take Back Day. https://www.deadiversion. usdoj.gov/ drug_disposal/takeback/. Last visited July 12, 2018.

6. NIH. National Institute of Drug Abuse. Overdose Death Rates Revised August 2018. https://www.drugabuse.gov/related-topics/trends- statistics/ overdose-death-rates. Accessed August 16, 2018.

7. Robert W. Patterson. Statement Before the House Judiciary Committee U.S. House of Representatives For a Hearing Entitled: "Challenges and Solutions in the Opioid Abuse Crisis" Presented on May 08, 2018 https:// www.dea.gov/pr/speeches-testimony/2018t/050818t.pdf. Last visited August 1, 2018.

8. Drug Enforcement Administration. Diversion Control Division. Title 21 United States Code (USC) Controlled Substances Act. Oct. 27, 1986. https://www.deadiversion.usdoj.gov/21cfr/21usc/813.htm. Accessed July 24, 2018.

9. SAMHSA Shares Latest Behavioral Health Data, Including Opioid Misuse. 10/12/2017. https://newsletter.samhsa.gov/2017/10/12/ samhsa-new-da- ta-mental-health-substance-use-including-opioids/. Last visited August 21, 2018

10. Proposed Aggregate Production Quotas for Schedule I and II Controlled Substances and Assessment of Annual Needs for the List I Chemicals Ephedrine, Pseudoephedrine, and Phenylpropanolamine for 2019. August 20, 2018. https://www.deadiversion.usdoj.gov/fed_regs/ quotas/2018/ fr0820.htm. Last visited August 21, 2018.

Part Two

PREVENTION AND TREATMENT FOR PATIENTS WHO USE AND ARE ADDICTED TO OPIOIDS

Chapter 6

The Impact of the Opioid Epidemic

The opioid epidemic is, indeed, a consequential problem that by all accounts is getting worse. As it is now, the impact has created one of the most significant crises in our modern era.

Many sectors are joining forces to combat this epidemic. Members of the scientific communities, politicians, medical healthcare and service personnel, healthcare insurance companies, and pharmaceutical companies (to name a few) appear to be on board at some level. But despite their efforts, the opioid epidemic continues to impact our society devastatingly, and at levels that have never been seen before. There are numerous publications ranging from media sound bites, documentaries, articles, books, and others; one cannot get away from the statistics and numbers that are cited in these discussions and articles that try to make the point of how impactful this crisis is. This book is no exception; therefore, you'll frequently see statistical numbers repeated. Hopefully, it will raise our consciousness of where we are now, and all of us will better understand the importance of everyone being on board to fight this opioid epidemic. The scientific evidence and statistics that exist today clearly support the conclusion that we are in one of the most significant epidemics of our generation, if not the most significant.

The CDC states that in 2016, the number of fatal overdoses involving opioids was five times higher than in 1999. Also, between 1999 and 2016, there were 632,000 deaths in total from drug overdoses. In most of these deaths, 66% involve opioids. Approximately 40% of all opioid deaths involved legal- prescription opioids such as OxyContin or oxycodone, hydrocodone, and morphine. Non-prescription illegal opioids such as heroin and IMF account for the majority of deaths. More than 115 people per day died from opioid overdoses in 2016.[1,2]

Comparing 2015 and 2016 data, overdose fatalities due to IMF more than doubled: from 9,580 to 19,413, respectively. For the same years, heroin deaths increased by nearly 20%, while that from legal painkillers increased by about 11%.

The opioid-epidemic problems have not improved significantly. Overdose deaths from IMF are outpacing other illegal opioids by far. It has become more available, cheaper and deadlier.[2,3] Another important, closely related and contributing factor is the almost parallel increase in non-opioid-drug overdose, which has increased by about four times between 1999 and the 2016.[6]

Despite increased awareness and efforts to address the opioid epidemic, the CDC reports that between the third quarter of 2016 and the third quarter of 2017, overdoses from opioids have increased by about 30%. This was documented by emergency rooms and hospitals across the United States. The Midwest had a 69.7% increase, followed by the West with 40.3%, the Northeast with 21.3%, Southwest with 20.2%, and Southeast with 14%.[4]

The projected estimated total deaths from all drugs related to an overdose in the year 2017 are over 72,000, with approximately 49,000 being opioid-related. Deaths from fentanyl and its analogs, primarily IMF, are expected to be about 30,000.[17]

There are, however, some positive trends with respect to **prescription opioids** that are worth noting; the new opioid misusers, the total number of opioid misusers, and patients with opioid use disorder have shown decreasing number from 2015 to 2017. Similarly, new heroin users and the total number of heroin users are down from the year 2016 to 2017. However, overdose deaths from heroin have continued to increase.[20]

The economic burden and healthcare costs continue to rise. The Institute of Medicine estimates that over 100 million Americans are suffering from chronic pain, costing the economy upwards of $635 billion per year. The Economic Advisory Council also estimated that in 2015, the costs to the economy due to deaths and overdoses related to the epidemic was $504 billion.[5,9]

The vast majority of these chronic pain patients are likely to consume opioids at some point. Some of them, if not treated appropriately, will become addicted to opioids and will become a statistic, in terms of both financial health and mortality. The health crisis caused by the opioid epidemic has created a significant financial burden on the country and the law enforcement budget, among others, and the healthcare system in particular. Increased costs related to crimes and law enforcement are needed to deal with associated drug-related incidents and/or trafficking.

The effect on families and their loved ones is immeasurable. So many have lost their lives to addiction. There are countless families that have been ripped apart, both emotionally and financially; their efforts or time spent to save their loved ones come to no avail.

Very often, when someone becomes an addict, that person is no longer capable of fully understanding the consequences of his or her actions, or even care about them anymore. They will do anything that will ensure their supply of drugs or opioids so they can satisfy their cravings.

The effect of the improper use and abuse of opioids will transform someone who is considered normal, and make them into someone with a disorder or addiction. At this point, that person has lost control of his or her life, and often of reality. Users who end up in this condition are no longer the person they used to be; therefore, normal approaches that usually work and generate a rational response from them will no longer apply. They will require professionals who can manage and deal with some of the most difficult problems and challenges anyone will ever face.

Children sometimes have nowhere to go after being taken into child custody and placed into foster homes or foster care. Occasionally, some capable and willing relatives will come to their aid and perform the duties of parents. This is necessary because their parents often are no longer available because of death or inability to care for their children.

Unfortunately, some babies or neonates are born with addiction: **Neonatal Abstinence Syndrome**. This is inherited from their mothers who weren't able or didn't want to stop using opioids during their pregnancy. Now, their babies are born addicted to opioids. They will go through opioid withdrawal, require treatment comparable to what adults require, and have to go to through detoxification.

Sometimes, these babies will be exposed to other associated drugs and will have developmental issues because of their mothers' use of multiple substances while pregnant. This adds to or complicates the recovery, growth, and often survival of the neonates. In addition, these babies will require an extended stay in neonatal intensive care units, adding to the financial burden of the opioid epidemic.

The economics of the opioid epidemic has a significant impact on the poor or underserved. This doesn't mean that wealthy or more affluent individuals are not affected. Everyone and anyone can be and are potential victims. You may not be directly involved, but by extension, your loved ones or relatives might be.[19]

However, it is important to mention that a part of the population that uses opioids, primarily those who do not obtain prescriptions legally from healthcare providers, find themselves at even more significant risk.

In general, there is a large number of users of opioids who cannot afford to obtain medical care or to obtain the services of counselors or other healthcare providers that will reduce their risk of addiction. These individuals often have the most challenging and difficult course in the process of recovery. They usually have minimal family or social support structures in place, and often have no finances or minimal finances. Also, they have no medical care or healthcare insurance to support the complex needs of their medical condition. It is not uncommon to see some of these users in and out of the criminal justice system; the worst-case scenario is that they have a higher probability and are more prone to fatal opioid overdoses.

Am I My Brother's Keeper?

Well, if I am my brother's keeper, who is my keeper? The opioid epidemic has serious consequences; and has ultimately led to an unprecedented increase in the number of deaths and destruction, particularly over the last 20 years. This question often arises: what can I do, as a family member, friend, loved one, or just someone who cares?

There are many challenges that must be faced. One of the biggest and most difficult ones is accepting the fact that someone that you care about is a drug abuser, possibly an addict.

This often presents itself with multiple denials, as well as shame and embarrassment in facing reality for which almost no one is prepared. However, as painful as that may be, it is even more painful to watch someone you care about being taken away from you… DEAD because of your failure to intervene at an appropriate time that might've made a significant difference.

The concept of looking out for one another is not new. Regardless of when it happens, once a person starts traveling down the path of drug abuse and addiction, that person is no longer the person they used to be. They usually have lost control of themselves and their ability to be rational and make sound decisions. In other words, their brains have been hijacked by their favorite drugs or substances, are literally structurally changed.[10,11,12]

Intervention is critically important before and during this period. It may be necessary to take very drastic action to save the life of the person you care about. Sometimes, it may involve law enforcement to put the person away for their own safety. One has to realize that love and compassion, although important in times like these, can only be beneficial if strong boundaries are established and followed. It is also very important to understand that if the users or your loved ones are in and out of drug rehab, or if from time to time they uses illegal drugs or abuses prescription drugs, they need to be watched, monitored and treated.

This means that family members, friends, and loved ones need to be active participants in each other's lives, or in the users' lives.

What Signs Should You Look Out For?

The privilege that we have as physicians and medical providers that is given to us by the DEA allows us to prescribed opioids, and controlled substances is one of the most significant responsibilities we have as healthcare providers. This fact seems to escape a significant number of healthcare providers probably because so many of us do have a license to prescribed opioids and controlled substances. In addition, most of us do not abuse or misuse our privilege to prescribe.

One of the critical facts to remember in prescribing opioids is that these medications create analgesic (pain reducing) effect by binding to receptors in the nervous system called "**mu-agonist receptors.**" The more we increase the dose of opioids the greater the effect of decreasing the amount of pain that individuals taking these medications will experience.

This means that there is no **ceiling effect** (*meaning there is no decrease in analgesic effect after a certain maximum dose of medication is reached*) in ingesting an increasing dose of opioids for pain reduction. The amount of opioids that each person consumes will be limited in part by the associated adverse effects from the escalating dose received or ingested. Therefore, **one may be experiencing very little or no pain and be dying at the same time** because of respiratory failure from the adverse effects of opioids shutting down his or her respiratory system.

It is therefore imperative that medical providers prescribing opioids (and also other controlled substances) realize how important it is to prescribe responsibly, he functional gatekeepers of how and when these medications are prescribed and how they are used. We can always find justifications in increasing patients' opioids, but we must bear in mind the adverse effects, the risks of developing (see below) opioid tolerance, physical dependence, addictions (opioid use disorder) and of course leading to opioid- related deaths.

For most people who are on low or minimum doses of legally prescribed opioid, not many changes or any can be identified initially. However, it is worth mentioning that an individual can get hooked on opioids with a minimal initial dose. The best option is always prevention.

Developing a Tolerance to Drugs

One of the first signs that develops is **tolerance**: this is a state where a previously prescribed dose of opioids or previously used illegal dose is not as effective as it used to be. Now, the user requires more or higher doses to control their pain or to gain the high/euphoria they are accustomed to. At this point, it is critical to have dedicated professionals who understand pain management and addiction to intervene and help manage the situation. The illegal user is, of course, at the greatest disadvantage because virtually anything goes.

Developing a Physical Dependence on Drugs

After tolerance, the next significant sign is **physical dependence**. This is a state where the discontinuation of medication results in withdrawal symptoms like nausea, vomiting, diarrhea, increased pain, and weakness. Usually, resumption of medication(s) or substance(s) improves or stops the symptoms.

This is really a very dangerous stage because the symptoms described above for tolerance may also be present for physical dependence. However, there are also early signs of drug-seeking behavior such as overtaking medications or using medications not prescribed by their medical providers. Users still have some control over their actions, are amenable to change with or without significant intervention, and may have no significant and lasting neuropsychological deficits once they're off the medications.

Intervention, often with a multidisciplinary or multimodal approach, is always preferred. This will also reduce the risks of significant withdrawals, which could lead to a more inappropriate indulgence, and even addiction if the dependency is not addressed professionally.

Developing Addiction or Substance Use Disorder

The next and worst stage is **addiction or substance use disorder**, or in the case of the opioid epidemic, **opioid use disorder**. At this point, the users are likely to have lost their ability to care about the consequence of their actions because of neurological changes that have occurred in their brain. They will be satisfied temporally so long as their drugs' requirements are met. They feel compelled to take whatever actions they deem necessary.

As above, the need for professionals who understand pain, addiction medicine, and other associated disciplines must be involved. These individuals tend to withdraw and develop a craving for their drugs of choice easily.

Their withdrawals are usually significant, and their cravings are pronounced. In simple neuropsychological and neurobiological terms, the circuits of their brain no longer function the way they should. In other words, there are physical, chemical and neuropsychological changes that have occurred, and transformed each addict or substance use disorder individual into a differentperson.

Therefore, stopping the drug abuse and going through extensive detoxification/drug rehabilitation does not restore the damage done to the brain. The journey to recovery will be long and often difficult and requires supportive care from professionals as well as loved ones.[11,13]

What about Opioid Drug Overdoses?

One of the most critical points in opioid use is the understanding that whether one is using legal drugs such as oxycodone, hydrocodone, or morphine; or illegal opioids such as heroin or IMF, *overdose can and will occur at any stage or any point during use of any of these drugs*.

There are undoubtedly some cases where overdoses are more likely than others — for example, those who have developed tolerance, physical dependence or addiction. However, ***one does not have to develop tolerance, dependence or addiction to have a drug overdose resulting in their death.***

Combining Drugs Can Kill You

Overdoses also occur more frequently and are more likely when certain other drugs are taken together with opioids. When one or more illegal drugs such as cocaine, methamphetamine, and marijuana are mixed and/or taken with opioids, deaths are more likely.

It is also extremely important is to avoid combinations of benzos (such Xanax, Valium, Ativan, etc.) and/or mix alcohol with opioids; any of these combinations can and often be deadly in many cases.[14,15,17]

Believing You Have a High Tolerance for a Large Amount of Drugs Can Kill You

Another important situation or scenario where overdose risk increases is when drug users or addicts are prevented from gaining access to the same amount of drugs their system is used to tolerating — for example, when they're incarcerated, or willfully stop or pause their drug use. It results in a state or condition where they are essentially cleared of drugs. In other words, they are clean and detoxed, even if that was not their intention.

Once the users decide to start using drugs again, they have a tendency to believe that they will be able to do the same amount as before. This falsehood often leads to a large number of previously high-dose users overdosing on a relatively modest or lower amount, often leading to death.

If a drug user or your family member or loved one was once a large-dose user of opioids and stopped using them for a period, and then decides to resume using those drugs at the same high level as before, be careful. The drug user's system will need some time to adjust before it can tolerate the high doses it was subjected before he or she stopped. He or she will be at a significantly increased risk of overdosing and dying from even smaller amounts than what was used before.[11,13]

Signs of Opioid Drug Use and/or Overdose

Awareness of the signs of drug use or overdose is often very helpful in allowing us to move with greater urgency. Some of the signs of drug use or overdose are as follows:

➢ The presence of drug paraphernalia

➢ Presence of syringes or needles

➢ Pills or pill bottle(s)

➢ Used drug containers – bags, cans, etc.

➢ Spoons or cookers

➢ Lighters

➢ Tourniquets, balloons, belts, etc.

➢ Modified smoking/inhalation pipes

Be aware of the symptoms of opioids overdose as well as withdrawal – please review these in section two of the book, under "Treatment" in Chapter 11.

Never Do Drugs Alone; Always Have Your Buddy with You

If you are your brother's keeper, or someone is your keeper, this is a simple but important concept to know: *I look out for you; you look out for me.*

ONE OF THE MOST IMPORTANT GOALS OF RECOVERING FROM OPIOID DEPENDENCE OR ADDICTION BEGINS WITH THE DISCONTINUATION OF THE SUBSTANCE THAT THE USERS WERE ABUSING — IN THIS CASE, OPIOIDS OR OTHER RELATED LEGAL OR ILLEGAL SUB- STANCES.

However, this book would not be complete without advising you or your caregiver or loved one always to ensure that no one does drugs alone. **This is by no means, an encouragement, endorsement or support of anyone to abuse drugs of any kind.**

The user should always be in the presence of someone they trust while shooting up/injecting, sniffing, smoking or swallowing or however the drugs are consumed. Both users should not be and must not be shooting up at the same time with the same drugs. One person needs to be available should something go wrong. *If one of the users overdoses and/or is dying,* **the survivor or awake person can possibly administer naloxone or summon help.**

This is the same concept that exists for swimming. No one should go swimming or diving alone, even if he or she has a pool in his or her backyard. That way, there is always someone to help in case one person gets into trouble. This means that doing drugs while locked away in one's room, basement or attic while others are in the house but are unaware of what he or she is doing does not prevent the user from dying. That person is still at extreme risk of dying from an overdose. The family members, loved ones or friends unaware of what is happening will be of no help despite the fact that they are so close.

Your Savior for Reversing an Overdose

<u>Naloxone,</u> also called Narcan, is a drug that will save lives if administered quickly and on time for an opioid overdose. This usually cannot be administered by the victims themselves, as they will likely be unconscious. Naloxone must be administered by a friend, family member, or anyone that has it ready to go when the need arises, particularly for addicts doing high doses.

Please review the usage instructions for naloxone in Chapter 11, under the "Treatment" section. Ensure that you understand and are capable of administering it or instructing others on how to do so.

References, Recommended Readings and Resources

1. Centers for Disease Control and Prevention. Understanding the Epidemic. https://www.cdc.gov/drugoverdose/epidemic/index.html.

2. Puja Seth, Ph.D.; Lawrence Scholl, Ph.D.; Rose A. Rudd, MSPH; Sarah Bacon, Ph.D., M*MMWR*. Overdose deaths involving opioids, cocaine, and psychostimulants – the United States, 2015 – 2016. https://www.cdc.gov/mmwr/volumes/67/wr/mm6712a1.htm. Accessed May 5, 2018.

3. U.S. drug overdose deaths continue to rise; increase fueled by synthetic opioids. https://www.cdc.gov/media/releases/2018/p0329- drug-overdose-deaths.html. Accessed May 5th, 2018.

4. Alana M. Vivolo-Kantor, Ph.D.; Puja Seth, Ph.D.; R. Matthew Gladden, Ph.D.; Christine L. Mattson, Ph.D.; Grant T. Baldwin, Ph.D.; Aaron Kite-Powell, MS; Michael A. Coletta, MPH Vital Signs: Trends in Emergency Department Visits for Suspected Opioid Overdoses — United States, July 2016–September 2017 *March 6, 2018,* MMWR. https://www.cdc.gov/mmwr/volumes/67/wr/mm6709e1.htm. Accessed June 17, 2018.

5. The Underestimated Cost of the Opioid Crisis. The Economic Advisory Council November 2017. https://www.whitehouse.gov/sites/ whitehouse.gov/files/images/The%20Underestimated%20Cost%20 of%20the%20Opioid%20Crisis.pdf. Accessed June 15, 2018.

6. NIH. National Institute on Drug Abuse. Opioid overdose Crisis. https://www.drugabuse.gov/drugs-abuse/opioids/opioid-overdose- crisis. Accessed June 4, 2018.

7. Drug Enforcement Administration. Drug Facts Sheet-Narcotics. https://www.dea.gov/druginfo/drug_data_sheets/Narcotics.pdf. Accessed July 4, 2018.

8. National Opioid Epidemic. amfAR, Opioid, and Healthcare Indicated Database. http://opioid.amfar.org/indicator/mme_percap. Accessed June 17, 2018.

9. Institute of Medicine. Relieving pain in America: a blueprint for transforming prevention, care, education, and research. Washington, DC: The National Academies Press; 2011. https://www. uspainfoundation.org/wp-content/uploads/2016/01/IOM-Full-Report. pdf. Accessed March 10, 2018.

10. Thomas Kosten, Tony P George. The Neurobiology of Opioid Dependence: Implications for Treatment. NIH. Science & Practice Perspectives. 13-20. August 2002. https://www.researchgate.net/ publication/5288549_The_Neurobiology_of_Opioid_Dependence_ Implications_for_Treatment. Accessed July 7, 2018.

11. National Institute on Drug Abuse. Principles of Drug Addiction Treatment: A Research-Based Guide. Third edition. Last reviewed December 2012. https://www.drugabuse.gov/sites/default/files/ podat_1.pdf. Accessed July 2, 2018.

12. George F. Koob. The neurobiology of addiction: a neuroadaptational view relevant for diagnosis. 08 August 006. https://onlinelibrary.wiley. com/doi/abs/10.1111/j.1360-0443.2006.01586.x. Accessed June 30, 2018.

13. George F Koob, Ph.D., Nora D Volkow, MD. Neurobiology of addiction: a neurocircuitry analysis. The Lancet Psychiatry. Volume 3, Issue 8, August 2016, Pages760-773. https://www.sciencedirect.com/ science/article/pii/S2215036616001048. Accessed on June 30, 2018.

14. Puja Seth, Ph.D.; Lawrence Scholl, Ph.D.; Rose A. Rudd, MSPH; Sarah Bacon, Ph.D., M*MMWR*. Overdose deaths involving opioids, cocaine, and psychostimulants – the United States, 2015 – 2016. https://www.cdc.gov/mmwr/volumes/67/wr/mm6712a1.htm. Accessed May 5, 2018.

15. Benzodiazepines and Opioids | National Institute on Drug Abuse (NIDA). March 2018. https://www.drugabuse.gov/drugs-abuse/ opioids/benzodiazepines-opioids. Accessed June 10, 2018.

16. Centers for Disease Control and Prevention (CDC). National Vital Statistics System, Mortality. CDC WONDER Online Database. https://wonder.cdc.gov/. Published 2017.

17. NIH. National Institute of Drug Abuse. Overdose Death Rates. https:// www.drugabuse.gov/related-topics/trends-statistics/overdose-death- rates. Accessed August 24, 2018.

18. National Institute on Drug Abuse. Principles of Drug Addiction Treatment: A Research-Based Guide. Third edition. Last reviewed December 2012. https://www.drugabuse.gov/sites/default/files/ podat_1.pdf. Accessed July 2, 2018.

19. Janet Currie and Molly Schnell. Harvard Business Review. A Closer Look at How the Opioid Epidemic Affects Employment. August 20, 2018. https://hbr.org/2018/08/a-closer-look-at-how-the-opioid-epidemic-affects-employment. Accessed August 20, 2018.

20. Reports and Detailed Tables From the 2017 National Survey on Drug Use and Health (NSDUH). https://www.samhsa.gov/data/nsduh/ reports-detailed-tables-2017-NSDUH Last accessed October 30, 2018.

Chapter 7

What Treatments are Available
Before Patients Become Addicted to Opioids?

In order to understand the available treatment options, it is relevant that each of us is aware of the various stages often involved in the treatment of pain that may lead to addiction. Of course, there is a significant number of individuals who become addicted to opioids and other controlled substances without ever having been treated for pain.

We will look at what typically happens when someone initially presents to a medical provider for pain treatment. We will examine the various paths of treatment protocols, as well as discuss how addiction may result from some of these initial treatments.

The general belief is that the overprescription of opioids is the root cause of the opioid epidemic. Also, two other factors contributed to this. The first occurred in about 2010, which saw a rapid increase in heroin overdose deaths; this was also the peak of opioid prescriptions' availability. The other is often referred to as the third phase; it began around 2013 when IMF was used in combination with heroin to produce a more potent drug cocktail.[1,2] We will also discuss those patients who became addicted without ever seeing a medical provider or any healthcare or social service personnel.

How Do We Treat Patients with Acute Pain and
Chronic Pain, but Have Never Used Any Significant Opioids?

In general, the approach that is best suited and advocated is a multidisciplinary or multimodal approach. This involves starting with non-opioids, gradually increasing these drugs, and subsequently adding short-acting opioids as opposed to long-acting or extended-release formulations. In addition, patients' psychosocial and behavioral history are taken into account and addressed. Wherever possible, coordination of care is incorporated with patients and family members as well as other providers.

The challenge, however, is that multidisciplinary or multimodal treatments are expensive and sometimes the people who need it most can't afford it or have healthcare insurance that offers only limited coverage. Also, a significant number of these patients tend to have poor psychosocial support.

Multiple non-opioids medication and therapeutic options are often used in the treatment of pain conditions often before opioids are introduced. These may include but are not limited to anti-inflammatory medication, non- narcotic analgesics, anti-spasmodic medication, and mood stabilizers. Patients may be required to be involved in physical therapy, psychiatric care, or behavioral therapy; or incorporate therapeutic modalities to enhance the treatment protocol.

The treatment protocol for pain, adapted for each patient, will vary depending on the chronicity or acuteness of the condition being treated, as well as the complexity of that condition and any other medical conditions (comorbidities) that may affect the treatment outcome. Numerous bodies/organizations such as the CDC, the US Department of Veterans Affairs, multiple medical associations and countless others have proposed and/or published treatment guidelines for patients that have acute and chronic pain.[3,4,5] In an effort to understand some of the content of this book as well as the various paths to recovery and/or addiction, we have included in **Appendix (E)** a flowchart (algorithm) called the **Foster's Opioid Classification Addiction Status (FOCAS)**.

Please take some time to review this and understand it, as it will make your reading more meaningful. Also refer to the **FOCAS TABLE**, which explains the flowchart that I will refer to from time to time. (It is not absolutely necessary for you to understand **FOCAS** to follow the discussion in this book). If you would like further details, you can find this flowchart and a detailed description in the book ***Foster's Opioid Classification Addiction Status Guide***, published by Global Health & Consortium Publishing in January 2019.

Treatments Available Before Patients Become Addicted to Opioids

Patients present to their healthcare providers very often with either acute pain or chronic pain. There is **acute pain,** defined as pain which will typically resolve in about three months; and **chronic pain,** which lasts longer than three months.

Acute pain may be the result of minor injuries, automobile accidents, workers compensation-related accident/injuries, and procedures such as surgeries by various specialists: orthopedic, dental, podiatry, etc. Others may have nonspecific pain, for example, in the stomach, ear, or headaches.

Patients with acute pain injuries and/or surgical procedures would fall into **Class 1: Groups 1 A, 1B and 1C** if they have never taken or have only used opioids minimally in the past (example: small quantities of opioids with a few days' duration, given by dentists and other specialists), or are so-called naïve patients. Depending on the severity of their injuries or procedures, they may be started on non-opioid medications as a first-line treatment, as recommended by the CDC guidelines and others.[3] However, some of these patients are started on opioids; again, this depends on the severity and type of injuries/procedures.

Other factors that dictate what these patients are started on are the medical providers and the treatment options they have available or are capable of administering. One could reasonably justify the need for opioids in someone who had an amputated limb as opposed to someone who sprained one of the joints in their extremity. The big questions are often: how long is it appropriate to continue opioids particularly for someone who has a significant injury, or underwent major surgery? Is a seven-day prescription enough, and if not, how much longer? And during that course, how much medication is considered appropriate?

Very often, the patients who did not respond to non-opioid therapeutic intervention would have continued on opioids and entered into the chronic phase of pain management.

The providers at this point will have to decide on whether or not they want to continue treating the patient and managing their opioids/pain management needs.

Patients in **Class 2: Groups 2A, 2B, and 2C** sometimes with minor injuries become chronic pain patients and, in some instances, would have been given more opioids than is appropriate. These patients would join the chronic opioid- naïve patients who have failed to respond to non-opioids or opioids in the initial phase of treatment.

It is worth mentioning that there are some other factors that sometimes cause some patients to go from acute status to chronic. Some of these patients may be involved in automobile accidents/personal injuries, workers' compensation injuries, and other litigation-pending injuries. Because of potential secondary gain and pending or unsettled cases, some of these patients may continue to take opioids even though their condition may not justify the need. Other patients who also may have secondary gains are patients who are on disability and need to "remain sick" in order to keep validating their disability status.

What Other Options are There Other Than Opioids Medications?

There is a wide range of non-opioid medications: some are anti-inflammatory, muscle relaxers, neuropathic, and for mood stabilization, wherever applicable. These are generally not addictive or have significantly less addictive potential than opioids. Some mood stabilizers are addictive and have similar risks factors to opioids.

The benefits of medications are often enhanced by a wide range of available ***none medication or limited medication options treatments****. Some of them are:*

➢ Physical Therapy

➢ Occupational Therapy

➢ Chiropractic Care

➢ Massage Therapy/Hydromassage therapy

➢ Yoga, Pilates, and Tai Chi

➢ Spinal Intervention Procedures (epidural, facets joint block, nerve block injections)

➢ Spinal Cord Stimulator Implementation

➢ Pain Pump Implementation

➢ Peripheral/Medial Branch Nerve/Stimulation

➢ Joint Injections (examples: knees and hips others)

➢ Muscular Injection – Trigger Points

➢ Biofeedback

➢ Cognitive Behavioral Therapy

➢ Regenerative Medicine – Platelet Rich Plasma (PRP)/Stem Cell Therapy

➢ Prolotherapy

➢ Psychotherapy

➢ Acupuncture/Acupressure

➢ Botox Injection – migraine headache

➢ Botox Injection - specificity treatment

➢ Non-Invasive Brain Stimulation – chronic pain

➢ Spinal Decompression Therapy

➢ Device Applications (examples: ultrasound, TENS unit, traction device, etc.) (by therapists/instructors).

A significant number of these options are very useful and can be an essential part or types of other treatment protocols for patients in the initial stage of opioid therapy. Some of them are also very important in complementing the treatments for patients with substance dependence, as well as opioid addiction.

Special Categories
Natural Products and Supplements

The treatment of pain can take on different courses dictated by the persons in pain, their culture, medical trends, and the limitations imposed by state or federal regulations, among other things.

The use of natural products and or supplements, as well as treatments classified as **Alternative Medicine (Complementary Medicine) Traditional Medicine**, often leads to vigorous debates among supporters of both **Alternative Medicine** and **Modern Medicine**. Basically, **Alternative Medicine** refers to practices and treatments that were done by different cultures, sometimes for generations.

In many instances, these are being practiced in a different part of the world today. **Modern Medicine (Western Medicine)** refer to medicine as we know it today: visiting our primary care doctors and getting medications from pharmaceutical companies intended to treat conditions like diabetes, blood pressure, pain, etc., (sometimes referred to as Traditional Medicine). Also, in this general category of Alternative and/or Complementary Medicine, the term Non-traditional Medicine is frequently used. These include treatments and protocols that are sometimes not considered the standard of modern medical care.

Treatment therapy may include but is not limited to, specialized massage therapy, acupuncture, tai chi, and the use of spices and herbs. However, sometimes some of the practices or treatments of Non-traditional Medicine or Alternative Medicine are becoming more commonly used as part of the protocols of Modern Medicine resulting in overlaps of the different types of medicine.

Some common compounds that are used to treat pain include:

**Cayenne Pepper, Turmeric, Ginger,
Boswellia, Moringa and Guinea Hen Weed.**

Cayenne Pepper: from this, **capsaicin cream or cayenne cream** is produced. It is believed to work by binding to compounds in the body called substance P, which is responsible in part for the pain we feel. Capsaicin 8% Patch is also available for a single-dose application that may be repeated every three months as needed.

Turmeric: from this, a compound called **curcumin** is identified, and believed to have significant anti-inflammatory properties that are helpful in relieving pain.

Ginger: this compound is also believed to have significant anticancer properties and can be used to treat pain. It may be used as a drink or vegetable.

Boswellia: also known as Indian frankincense, known for its anticancer properties and widely used as such.

Moringa: often considered one of those herbs that have many different properties for treating many different conditions. Often used for anti- inflammatory properties concerning pain.

Guinea Hen Weed: known for its multiple effects on different medical conditions. It is also believed to have anti-inflammatory properties useful for treating painful conditions.

Kratom: also called Mitragnya Speciosa, tropical plants that are commonly found in Asia – for example, in Thailand and Malaysia. It is often used in the form of pills or powder or tea. It is believed to contain many compounds, some of which have similar properties to that of opioids. Also, its properties are believed to be similar to psychoactive compounds like LSD and PCP. Some patients use it for pain control as well as anxiety, depression and even treatment for opioid withdrawal.

Kratom has been in use in Asia for many years for similar treatments. The FDA considers kratom and its compounds to be opioids, essentially. This means that it or its components have the same ability and/or functions that traditional opioids have. Hence, its potential for abuse, use, misuse, and addiction are considered similar.

The DEA had considered classifying it as a Schedule I compound. However, this was delayed primarily due to significant opposition from its users and supporters of its uses and ongoing research. It still remains unclassified with respect to schedule by the DEA. However, there are few states that have banned the use of kratom.[7,8]

It is not without overdose and deaths being attributed to its use, in addition, like all other drugs, its users will continue to create their own cocktails, which often can be dangerous or deadly. However, kratom is still very popular and even has its own organization. The American Kratom Association is a strong advocate for its continued use.

Note on General Supplements/Vitamins

Multivitamins and minerals have always been seen as beneficial when taken appropriately. The general belief is that anything that optimizes the overall functioning of the body will ultimately lead to less pain and better well-being.

There are many in the field of medicine that advocate the use of multivitamins and their beneficial effects. Vitamins B and D are usually the common ones that many people believe are essential for well-being.

The use of minerals such as calcium, selenium, zinc, and magnesium; as well as compounds such as omega-3 fatty acids have been associated with better maintenance and/or development of muscle and bones as well as general well-being.

There are many publications that also encourage the use of alkaline water and low-sugar or no-sugar consumption; these are often helpful in creating a healthier and pain-free body. Now, some of these are considered unproven, or without a significant scientific basis for their use. However, there is a significant number of people engaged in alternative or complementary medicine. They are simply looking at non-traditional medicine for whatever condition that they may have as opposed to our traditional or modern medicine approach to the treatment of illness. In non-traditional or alternative medicine, the general approach is prevention, which usually leads to fewer illnesses and more effective treatments

The traditional medicine or modern medicine approach is the treatment of illness as the primary focus of therapeutic intervention rather than prevention.

Caution on the Use of Supplements, Natural Products, and Herbs

The inclusion of substance and/or compounds in this book should not be taken as an endorsement for their use. The descriptions here are purely for informational purposes. This will also enhance your awareness of their availability. In addition, upon completing your own research and consulting with your medical doctor, you will determine whether or not any of these is suitable for you.

It is also very important for everyone to understand that natural products/ vitamins and minerals have a minimum standard they have to meet for them to be sold to the public. There are no strict requirements; for example, these products are not pharmaceutical-grade like those prescribed and used for blood pressure, diabetes, etc. This means almost anyone can conceivably make and sell these products and, with skillful labeling and marketing, can sell it to the general public legally.

Also remember that with most natural products, the consistency, amount and purity are often very difficult to maintain and control at an appropriate and consistent level. This means that whatever response you received today may vary from treatment to treatment, even though in theory, you are taking the same recommended amount.

Always remember that if you are taking or plan to take any of these products, consult your primary care physicians/healthcare providers and ensure that you have significantly reduced the risks of experiencing unintended consequences or interactions with your other prescribed medications.

The Often Overlooked State of Well-Being

There is a direct or indirect correlation between almost everything we do and the effect it has on our well-being. Our bodies at some point were close to being perfect, or already were perfect. However, we change that with what we eat, the level of physical activity we engage in, the things we feed our mind, our spiritual being as we see fit to express or don't express, and so many other factors or triggers we allow to impact our lives.

The concept of pain or the theory of pain and how our bodies respond is not separate from all these things. Therefore, as each of us dictates how we live, we challenge our minds to determine who we are, what we continue to be, and ultimately, how we feel. This also leads us to the level of spirituality or openness we have in our lives.

If your body is not well, not only will the pain be part of your life, it can literally control it and take you to places no one should ever be. So, part of improving or decreasing the amount of pain you have is to strive to be well in all the facets of your lives.

Of course, this means eliminating smoking or tobacco use from our lives, as well as illicit or illegal drugs and substances such as alcohol that is toxic to our bodies. It is important also to exercise, ensure that that the diet you consume is right for your body and your weight is appropriate. Moreover, **after consulting with your healthcare providers**, remove some of your legally prescribed medications from your daily lives, whenever it is appropriate to do so.

References, Recommended Readings and Resources

1. Gery P. Guy Jr., Ph.D.; Kun Zhang, Ph.D.; Michele K. Bohm, MPH; Jan Losby, Ph.D.; Brian Lewis; Randall Young, MA; Louise B. Murphy, Ph.D.; Deborah Dowell, MD. CDCMMWR. Vital Signs: Changes in Opioid Pre- scribing in the United States, 2006–2015. July 7, 2017 / 66(26);697-704. https://www.cdc.gov/mmwr/volumes/66/wr/mm6626a4.htm?s_cid=m- m6626a4_w. Accessed March 1,2018.

2. The Centers for Disease Control and Prevention. Understanding the Epidemic. https://www.cdc.gov/drugoverdose/epidemic/index.html. Last visited June 16, 2018.

3. Deborah Dowell, MD; Tamara M. Haegerich, Ph.D.; Roger Chou, MD. CDC Guideline for Prescribing Opioids for Chronic Pain — the United States, 2016. March 18, 2016. https://www.cdc.gov/mmwr/ volumes/65/rr/ rr6501e1.htm. Accessed March 7,2018.

4. VA/DoDClinical Practice Guideline for Opioid Therapy for Chronic Pain. Department of Veterans Affairs Department of Defence. February 2017.https:// www.healthquality.va.gov/guidelines/Pain/cot/VADoDOTCPG022717. pdf. Accessed March 7,2018.

5. National Institute on Drug Abuse. Principles of Drug Addiction Treatment: A Research-Based Guide. Third edition. Last reviewed December 2012. https://www.drugabuse.gov/sites/default/files/ podat_1.pdf. Accessed July 2, 2018.

6. D. Terrence Foster. Foster's Opioid Classification Addiction Status. Global Health Consortium Publishing. January 2019. (If you would like further details, you can find this flowchart in that book)

7. Nick Wing. Kratom Users in States That Ban It Discuss How Prohibition Has Made Life Worse. 06/25/2018. https://www.huffingtonpost.com/entry/ kratom-ban-states_ us_5b2bc298e4b00295f15a3b83. Accessed June 29, 2018.

8. Peter Hess. The House Just Passed a Bill That Could Make Kratom Illegal. June 18, 2018. https://www.inverse.com/article/46088-what- is- the-sitsa- act-and-what-does-it-mean-for-kratom. Accessed June19, 2018.

Chapter 8

Is Marijuana… Cannabis the Last Hope?

Cannabis—a.k.a. Marijuana, Hemp, Ganja, Weed, Hashish, Pot: A Category on Its Own

I chose a special subcategory for cannabis because it is one of those substances, compounds or herbs which has generated significant interest for many different reasons.[1] In this book, I've chosen to use marijuana and cannabis interchangeably, although strictly speaking, marijuana refers to the dry leaves and flowers of the cannabis plant. The name "marijuana" is generally more common in most of the world and tends to generate more emotions than cannabis. Marijuana is also considered the most commonly used illegal drug around the world.[24]

I have also referred to marijuana as illegal. If you live in one of about 31 states plus the District of Columbia and counting in the United States where medicinal marijuana is decriminalized, or the eight states and the District of Columbia and counting where it is almost completely legal (including for recreational uses), then you probably wonder what I am talking about.

What I'm talking about is this: **marijuana, with respect to the federal laws of the United States, is illegal in all 50 states and the District of Columbia except for approval research settings**. This fact does not prevent states from enacting their own laws and regulations regarding marijuana use.

Cannabis (also called marijuana) is an herbal plant with many compounds that can potentially be extracted, called cannabinoids. In addition to cannabinoids, there also compounds called flavonoids and terpenoids or terpenes. These are the active compounds or chemicals that create the effects of marijuana. They are believed to be responsible for marijuana's therapeutic and/or medicinal properties. Some of these cannabinoids, flavonoids, and terpenoids may also be responsible for undesirable symptoms and signs that may manifest when marijuana is used or when one becomes intoxicated from its use.[2]

There are estimated to be more than 100 different cannabinoids that have already been extracted and identified. Some of these are more well-known and more studied than others. There are various wide-ranging estimates of the number of compounds. Some estimates put the number at about 400 different compounds in addition to the cannabinoids.[23]

The cannabinoids are believed to have their effects on our bodies by acting on the body's natural endocannabinoid system, which has its own cannabinoids, neurotransmitters, and receptors regulating the body's physiological processes. These may include but are not limited to pain, sleep, mood or appetite.

Delta-9 Tetrahydrocannabinol (THC)

The most commonly extracted and well-known cannabinoid from marijuana is THC (Delta-9 Tetrahydrocannabinol), which in some instances may represent about 30% of the compounds found in marijuana. However, the amount of THC does vary and may be as little as less than 1%. This is often determined by the strain of plants, and where and how they were cultivated, among other factors.

THC is more often considered responsible for the high or psychoactive effects experienced by marijuana users. These may include, but are not limited to the feeling of euphoria or feeling high, the lack of inhibitions, visual hallucinations, and decreased concentration. Its use in treatment has also been credited with an improvement in patients with pain due to its strong anti-inflammatory and muscle relaxant effects. It is also believed to have possible beneficial effects for seizures, Alzheimer's, and even some forms of cancer.

Cannabidiol (CBD)

Also, present in a significant amount from marijuana extracts is CBD (cannabidiol). The level of CBD found in marijuana is generally low. However, this depends on the strain, and how it was cultivated.[3] CBD has been extracted from the hemp plant, often referred to as industrial cannabis or hemp. Hemp usually has the highest percentage of CBD and a minimal amount or percentage of THC. The extraction of CBD oil is usually done from the leaves, flowers, and stalks. The percentage of CBD may range from less than 1% to about 10%. Because of the low THC percentage (usually less than 0.3%), the CBD oil produced from hemp plants are legal in all 50 states and the District of Columbia. It is therefore sold as supplements and in stores and via the internet. In general, cannabis products such as CBD oil with less than 0.3% THC are considered legal under federal and state laws.

The seed of the hemp plants is also used to produce hemp oil. The seeds and stalks are also used to make various products ranging from supplements, body care, household products, and others. However, consumers need to be aware, as there are many companies that market and sell "CBD oil" and other related marijuana products that, when tested, often aren't as advertised. Another problem concerns the conditions indicated for use, such as different illnesses that have not been approved by the FDA or any relevant scientific research.[4]

Charlotte's Web is a proprietary hemp-extracted product, which extracts CBD from hemp plants. The cannabis-hemp plants are cultivated to produce specific strains from which the CBD oil is extracted. This is believed to be the highest percentage of CBD available – about 20% compared to only about THC's 0.3% content. Therefore, because of the very low THC's content, the psychoactive effects usually associated with it should be minimum to none for individuals using Charlotte's Web. This product is primarily used to treat epileptic seizures and has reported success.[5,6,9,26]

It is also very important to remember that although THC and CBD are often talked about, other cannabinoids, terpenoids, and flavonoids are usually part of the extracted products that are commonly sold or available for use.

There are CBD oil products other than Charlotte's Web that are used to treat seizures. Most of them are extracted from hemp plants. The CBD content or percentage of extracts will be often determined by the strain that is produced, and how it is produced. That is, how much CBD versus THC is present will also determine how it is marketed and whether it can be sold legally; it depends on the percentage of THC present, required to be 0.3% or less.[5,6]

CBD and THC have been found to be beneficial in pain relief which is attributed to their anti-inflammatory effects. Other important possible benefits of CBD are: it is believed to decrease anxiety, and used to treat nausea and vomiting, Alzheimer's and Parkinson's disease, blood pressure or diabetes, among others.[9]

Extractions of THC and CBD

With regard to the extractions of THC and CBD, various methods are available. Some involve solvent extraction such as using propane, alcohol, butane, carbon dioxide or other solvents. The purity of the end products of cannabinoids rich in THC or CBD will depend on how the extractions are done and the type of solvents used. Extraction may also be accomplished by distillation, considered among the purest forms of separation or the concentration of products.

Products rich in THC or CBD may serve lots of beneficial purposes; but have the potential for deleterious effects, depending on how these very potent and concentrated compounds are used.[7]

Some other cannabinoids, including Marinol (dronabinol) and Cesamet (nabilone), are used to treat or prevent nausea and vomiting in cancer patients undergoing chemotherapy. These drugs are approved by the US FDA for the treatment indicated. Although marijuana has shown promise in treatment in laboratory studies, it is not approved by the FDA for treating cancer in humans. Marijuana is one of the most heavily researched herbal plants.

There are ongoing researches looking at the various aspects and different uses of the cannabinoids, flavonoids, and terpenoids found in these plants. Many requests to the DEA have been made to reclassify marijuana from Schedule I to Schedule II. This is advocated based in part on the amount of research results available and what many considered to be relatively less adverse side effects and medical benefits compared to other medications/substances in Schedule I and II groups. However, these requests have been denied multiple times, and marijuana remains illegal under federal laws, except for approved research settings.

Various studies have shown marijuana to be possibly effective in the treatment of noncancer and chronic pain, as well as cancer-related pain. There also studies that show the opposite. There are many other conditions for which cannabinoids have been found to be useful or advocated. Some of these uses do have strong support in the literature, while others are strongly refuted.

Also, in some of these researches, the response one gets from marijuana use may be dependent on how it is ingested: by smoking, vaporizing (inhaled), or orally (sprayed under the tongue). How you take it or ingest it might determine the response you get for the condition that you are trying to treat.

The debates over the use of cannabis or marijuana is an ongoing one, and it will continue for a long time. Clearly, it has medicinal benefits and the potential for abuse and misuse. One could also reasonably argue that the same applies to many pharmaceutical drugs or alcohol, which have significantly greater risks and potential for their abuse and misuse. But make no mistake about it: marijuana is a very complex plant, with many compounds and or chemicals contained in one product. There are over 100 cannabinoids. Some reports say it has about 400 flavonoids, terpenoids and other compounds whose numbers are unknown. Also unknown are the properties and functionalities of the intrinsic compounds, some of which are yet identified or studied. This makes the chemistry of marijuana very fascinating, to say the least. The idea to identify, and possibly design and construct, compounds will be and must be enjoyed by most researchers in this field. There are simply almost no limits on where this can go.

With respect to marijuana and the opioid epidemic, several publications and or studies have shown a positive trend with respect to decreasing the use of opioids in states where marijuana is legal for medicinal/recreational use. Two recent studies have shown that in part: "medicinal cannabis laws are associated with a significant reduction in opioids prescribing in the Medicare Part D population."[11]

The second study found that there was a 5.88% lower rate of opioid prescriptions in states that implemented medicinal marijuana laws.[10] These results can be considered positive trends with respect to the use or legalization of marijuana. Also, in general, they may be signals that probably indicate a potential way or option that could have an impact on reducing opioids use.

There are also other publications which revealed in part that in some states where marijuana is legal for medicinal/recreational use there is an increase in marijuana-related motor vehicle accidents fatalities as well as an increase in the use of marijuana as a gateway drug to other drugs such as cocaine and other illegal drugs.[29]

The Canadian Government And Cannabis

The Canadian government passed a bill to legalize cannabis nationally for recreational and of course medicinal use on June 18, 2018. This bill became law in October 2018 and is fully supported by the current prime minister. Canada is now one of the first major countries to fully legalize cannabis.[14,15,28]

Several American states have legalized cannabis for recreational use as well as medical purposes. However, as indicated, it is not legalized by the federal government in any state.

If you are physicians or medical providers, it is important that you realize your DEA license is given by the federal government, which will dictate how you can use it. This applies to all providers, regardless of which states we are practicing medicine in. Because of this, some physicians have chosen not to prescribe medicinal marijuana at all. In addition, they do not treat patients who have illegal drugs (including but not limited to cocaine, LSD and of course marijuana) in their system with simultaneously prescribed opioids or controlled substances. Sometimes, decisions have to be made when patients present with what is presumably legally obtained CBD oil or prescribed Marinol (an isomer of THC), a synthetic cannabinoid.

Therefore, both compounds will test positive for THC just as marijuana will. Providers then have to decide whether they are comfortable providing treatment, that is, prescribing opioids to patients who may be using both regular marijuana and any of the compounds which most probably will be positive for THC.

Several news media outlets, including the Wall Street Journal and Bloomberg News, reported the approval by the **FDA** of a compound called **Epidiolex, which is synthesized from CBD**.[12,13] This is the first FDA- approved medicinal use of the naturally occurring extract from marijuana for treating severe forms of childhood epilepsy, made by GW Pharmaceuticals PLC. *This is a significant development, which naturally leads to the following question: will marijuana still be considered to have no medical benefits when the FDA and DEA have now approved a significant component of it for medicinal use?* These same agencies use the "no medicinal benefits" line as part of their criteria to classify marijuana as Schedule I.

Now there are synthetic forms of THC available that the FDA has already approved, such as Marinol, Syndros, and Cesamet, which in part are attributed to the negative psychoactive effects associated with marijuana.

Marinol and Syndros are similar in structure to dronabinol, while Cesamet is similar in structure to **nabilone**. All three are used to treat nausea and vomiting associated with chemotherapy. Marinol and Syndros are also used to treat loss of appetite or anorexia.

The challenge of extracting significant enough quantities of identifiable compounds from marijuana has always been difficult because of a large number of different compounds. Therefore, it is generally difficult to obtain quantities large enough for research, testing and, ultimately, marketing at a commercial level. It is more realistic to anticipate the identification of components and then to synthesize the components or analogs (or isomers) of those compounds, hoping that they will have similar properties to what the extracted compounds have. However, this process is extremely challenging at different points.

On an almost positive note for marijuana research, several news agencies have reported that the DEA will or plan to authorize an increase in the production of marijuana by about fivefold: from about 1,000 pounds this year to over 5,000 pounds beginning in 2019. This would be the largest amount allowed in the history of marijuana production for research in the United States.[19,22]

However, we had heard the reverse of this occurring only in year 2017 when a small reduction in production was proposed. This is a dynamic issue, looking back at 2015, there was an increase that was proposed and effected.[20,21]

On the other hand, the DEA has an active Domestic Cannabis Eradication/ Suppression Program (DCE/SP) designed in part to eradicate and suppress marijuana cultivation that is not authorized for research by the federal government, as well as seize property related to cultivating and/or trafficking marijuana.

Marijuana is considered the only major abused drug grown within our borders. The DEA has a nationwide law enforcement program that exclusively targets drug trafficking organizations believed to be involved in marijuana production.[18]

My final two thoughts on marijuana:

1. If you believe in smoking or using marijuana the whole plant (without extracting each compound for its specific use), it is important you know that it is almost equivalent to having a bowl of probably about 500 very tiny pills. Most of their effects are unknown or unidentified; and some of them are known, as discussed above. Once you ingest this bowl of pills on any given day, God knows what you are taking. There's simply no standardize dosing for the use of marijuana.

2. In 2015, despite the fact that over 52,000 people died from drug overdose, the total number of deaths from marijuana was believed to be zero.[16,17]
   In addition, marijuana is now available in so many different edible forms, including oils, butter, cakes, and brownies. In general, there is no lethal dose for marijuana, but its users can become intoxicated and exhibit all or some of the adverse psychoactive and/or other symptoms that are associated with overdose.

   Another key factor in the use of marijuana is that there has been a significant increase in additives or compounds being added to "pure marijuana" making it even more unsafe than its natural form. This is often done to improve its potency or enhance the effects it has on its users. This of course has the potential for catastrophic consequences even leading to deaths.

If you are confused after reading this, don't worry you are among many.
Keep searching for knowledge.[25,29]

References, Recommended Readings and Resources

1. National Cancer Institute. Cannabis and Cannabinoids (PDQ®)– Patient Version.https://www.cancer.gov/about-cancer/treatment/cam/ patient/cannabis-pdq. Accessed March 30, 2018

2. Most Commonly Used Addictive Drugs. https://www.drugabuse.gov/ publications/media-guide/most-commonly-used-addictive-drugs. Last visited June 26, 2018.

3. National Institute on Drug Abuse. Commonly abused drugs charts. https://www.drugabuse.gov/drugs-abuse/commonly-abused-drugs- charts. Accessed April 2, 2018.

4. Thomas H. Clarke. FDA Issues Warnings to Makers of 'Legal'CBD Hemp Oil Products. March 8, 2015. http://www.thedailychronic. net/2015/41401/ fda-issues-warnings-to-makers-of-legal-cbd-hemp- oil-products/. Last visited July 10, 2018

5. The complete guide to concentrates. https://potguide.com/guides/ cannabis-concentrate-guide/. Accessed April 6, 2018.

6. Morgan Smith. Cannabis Distillate: Everything You Need to Know. January 6, 2017. https://potguide.com/pot-guide-marijuana-news/ article/canna- bis-distillate-everything-million grant from you-need-to- know/. Accessed April 6, 2018.

7. The Health Effects of Cannabis and Cannabinoids: The Current State of Evidence and Recommendations for Research (2017). Chapter: 4 Therapeutic Effects of Cannabis and Cannabinoids Therapeutic Effects of Cannabis and Cannabinoids. https://www.nap.edu/read/24625/ chapter/6#93. Accessed April 7, 2018

8. Cannabis 101: Charlotte's Web vs. Hemp Seed Oil versus Marijuana. February 7, 2017. https://www.cwhemp.com/blog/difference-hemp- marijuana. Last visited April 7, 2018.

9. Charlotte's web (cannabis). From Wikipedia, the free encyclopedia. ttps://en.wikipedia.org/wiki/Charlotte%27s_web_(cannabis). Last visited April 7, 2018.

10. Hefei Wen, Ph.D.; Jason M. Hockenberry, Ph.D. Association of Medical and Adult-Use Marijuana Laws with Opioid Prescribing for Medicaid Enrollees. JAMA Intern Med. 2018;178(5):673-679. May 2018. https://jamanet-work.com/journals/jamainternalmedicine/article- abstract/2677000. Accessed June 26, 2018.

11. Ashley C. Bradford, BA; W. David Bradford, Ph.D.; Amanda Abraham, Ph.D.; et al. Association Between US State Medical Cannabis Laws and Opioid addicted Prescribing in the Medicare Part D Population. *JAMA In- tern ed.* 2018;178(5):667-672. https://jamanetwork.com/journals/jamaint- ernalmedicine/article- abstract/2676999. Accessed June 26, 2018.

12. Anna Edney. Bloomberg. First Marijuana-Based Medicine Is Approved for Sale in U.S. June 25, 2018, https://www.bloomberg. com/news/articles/2018-06-25/first-marijuana-based-medicine-wins- approval-for-sale- in-u-s. Last visited July 27, 2018.

13. Peter Loftus. The Wall Street Journal. FDA Approves First Drug Derived from Marijuana Plant. June 25, 2018. https://www.wsj. com/articles/fda- approves-first-drug-derived-from-marijuana- plant-1529954791. Last visited July 27, 2018.

14. Monique Scotti. National Online Journalist, Politics Global News Marijuana legalization Bill C-45 officially passes Senate vote, heading for royal assent. June 19, 2018. https://globalnews.ca/news/4282677/ pot-bill-senate-passes/. Accessed June 20, 2018.

15. Peter Zimonjic. CBC News. Senate passes pot bill, paving the way for legal cannabis in 8 to 12 weeks. June 19, 2018. https://www.cbc.ca/ news/politics/senate-passes-government-pot-bill-1.4713222.Accessed June 20, 2018

16. Annual Causes of Death in the United States. http://www. drugwarfacts. org/chapter/causes of death. Accessed July 4,2018.

17. Rose A. Rudd, MSPH; Puja Seth, Ph; Felicita David, MS;Lawrence Scholl, Ph.D. Increases in Drug and Opioid-Involved Overdose Deaths — United States, 2010–2015. December 16, 2016. https://www.cdc.gov/mmwr/volumes/65/wr/mm655051e1.htm. Accessed July 4,2018.

18. DEA. Cannabis Eradication Domestic Cannabis Eradication / Suppression Program. https://www.dea.gov/cannabis-eradication. Accessed August

19. Tom Angell. DEA Wants More Marijuana Grown and Fewer Opioids Produced In 2019. Really. August 16, 2018. https://www.forbes.com/ sites/ tomangell/2018/08/16/dea-wants-more-marijuana-grown-and- fewer-opioids-produced-in-2019-really/#4e967b6c14cb. Accessed August 19, 2018

20. Alicia Wallace. DEA plans to reduce quota of government-grown marijuana for research in 2018. August 8, 2017. https://www. thecannabist. co/2017/08/08/dea-marijuana-research-quota-2018- nida/85321/. Accessed August 19,2018.

21. Oscar Pascual. DEA allows massive increase in marijuanaproduction (for research). June 17, 2015. http://sfevergreen.com/dea-allows- massive-in- crease-in-marijuana-production-for-research/. Accessed August 19, 2018.

22. Chris Moore. The DEA Plans to Grow More Weed for Scientific Research in 2019. August 17, 2019. https://merryjane.com/news/ the-dea-plans- to-grow-more-weed-for-scientific-research-in-2019. Accessed August 19, 2018.

23. The United States Drug Enforcement Administration. Learn the facts about Cannabis. https://www.dea.gov/taxonomy/term/336. Last visited August 21, 2018.

24. CBS/AP. Study: Marijuana is most popular illegal drug worldwide. August 29, 2013.https://www.cbsnews.com/news/study-marijuana-is-most-popular illegal drug-worldwide/. Accessed September 23, 2018.

25. The Institute for Behavior and Health. https://www.ibhinc.org/news/ Accessed October 29, 2018.

26. Dr. Sanjay Gupta, Full CNN Documentary Weed Part 4. April 30, 2018. https://www.youtube.com/watch?v=R90JW1fTw8U. Accessed September 23, 2018.

27. TroyTravels. CNN Dr. Sanjay Gupta Marijuana and Charlotte's Web. March 12, 2017. https://vimeo.com/207997748. Accessed September 23, 2018.

28. Darran Simon and Nicole Chavez Canada just legalized recreational pot. Here's what you need to know. October 17, 2018, https://www. cnn. om/2018/10/17/health/canada-legalizes-recreational-marijuana/index. html Accessed October 23, 2018.

29. Shannon M. Nugent, PhD; Benjamin J. Morasco, PhD; Maya E. O'Neil, PhD; Michele Freeman, MPH; Allison Low, BA; Karli Kondo, PhD; Camille Elven, MD; Bernadette Zakher, MBBS; Makalapua Motu'apuaka, BA; Robin Paynter, MLIS; Devan Kansagara, MD, MCR. The Effects of Cannabis Among Adults With Chronic Pain and an Overview of General Harms: A Systematic Review. 5 in September 2017.. *http://annals.org/aim/fullarticle/2648595/ effects-cannabis-among- adults-chronic-pain-overview-general- harms-systematic* Accessed September 23, 2018.

Free Useful Marijuana Information Brochures

Free useful brochures from NIDA with information in question-and-answer format about marijuana.

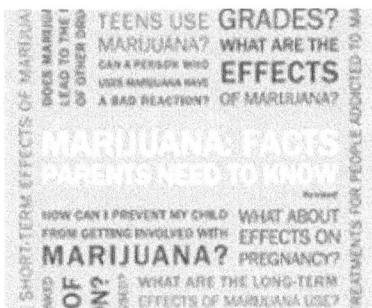

Marijuana: Facts Parents Need to Know

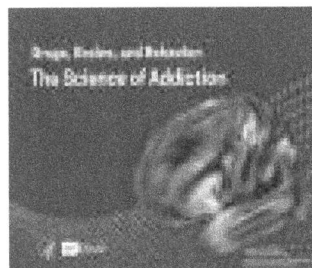

Mind Over Matter: The Brain's response to Marijuana

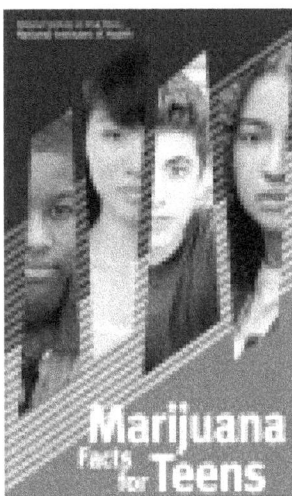

Facts for Teens

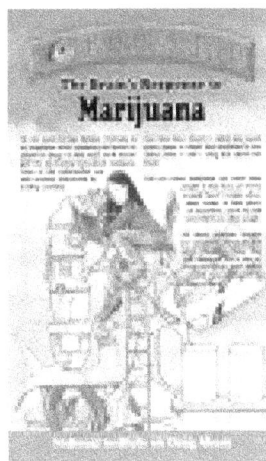

Drugs, Brains, and Behavior: The Science of Addiction

Call: 1-877-NIDA-NIH (1-877-643-2644)
or 1-240-645-0228 (TDD)

Fax: 1-240-645-0227   *Hours of operation: 8:30am–5:00pm ET*

View these publications online at: www.drugabuse.gov
National Institute of Drug Abuse
https://drugpubs.drugabuse.gov/publications/marijuana-facts-parents-need-know
Last accessed December 19,2018.

Chapter 9

What Treatment are Available after Patients Become Addicted to Opioids?

When Patients Become Chronic Users of Opioids

The vast majority of patients that have become chronic pain patients in their early stages were treated by primary care, family practitioners, internal medicine practitioners and, to a lesser extent, surgical specialists.

In general, over 50% of the opioids prescribed in the United States are prescribed by primary care physicians, family practices, and internal medicine physicians or providers.[1] Sometimes, it might be years before some of these patients are referred to **pain management specialists**. At that stage, they are either in **Class 3 or 4** and in some instances, heading into **Class 5**.

The challenges faced by some of these treating physicians/providers is that they either have limited options to offer pain patients other than medications, or they have additional options but failed to use them.

On the other hand, when patients present to pain specialists on high-dose opioids, they expect to have a similar treatment as they did with their primary care providers. Often, once this desire is not fulfilled, they are either discharged because of being noncompliant, or they leave on their own accord to go "shopping" to meet their opioid needs. Eventually, they are likely to get to a point where no one is able or willing to prescribe the amount of opioids they need, so they then end up seeking supplementation from illegal drugs like heroin and illicit synthetic opioids analogs. This often causes a downward spiral course if intervention and treatment are not initiated in a timely and aggressive manner.

Treatment of the Other 60% – Users of Illegal
Opioids such as IMF, its Synthetic Analogs, Heroin, and Others

Sixty percent of all opioid-related overdose deaths are directly related to users of illegal opioids such as heroin and IMF. Approximately 40% of opioid-related deaths are due to legally prescribed opioids.

Users of illegal opioids fall into three broad groups in **Class 5**, classified as **Group 5XA**, **5XB**, and **5XC**. Members of these groups usually function or operate without any or very limited healthcare, social services, or direct medical care or supervision. Sometimes, if any service is available, it probably is unrelated to their opioid substance abuse or needs.

Group 5XA: these are individuals who have no medical problem in general, and are simply using drugs for personal use or just experimenting. This group has the lowest average age, often comprised of teenagers and young adults. They may have obtained the opioid from someone's medicine cabinets, or through a friend, usually given free in the first few instances. They may also have received their first taste of opioids from cheap, available illegal heroin or IMF. This may have simply started as "I'll just try this; it'll make me feel better." Or "I have got something for you." This can and will often lead to the unaware, and unsuspecting users becoming addicted to the opioids or, even in the early introduction stage, lead to death by overdose.

This group of users often surprise their family and loved ones because they are generally considered "the best of society": everything to gain, and nothing to lose. However, once this naïve user of illegal opioids becomes addicted, and the free supply of legally prescribed opioids or illegal opioids are no longer available for free, then these victims become slaves to their opioid craving, "dependence/ addiction" and to their suppliers.

Group 5XB: these are individuals who do have a medical problem involving chronic pain without psychiatric disorders or other illegal substance abuse. They have failed to continue to get medical care because they don't have healthcare insurance or have noncompliance issues with previous legally prescribed pain management providers.

They now resort to obtaining medications from diversions; and once that is unavailable, they will resort to less expensive illegal drugs such as heroin or IMF or designer/analog drugs, presumably opioids. These patients generally may fall within the range of opioid tolerance to full-blown opioid addicts. Group 5XC: the users in this group are comprised of patients who have a history of or have developed mental disorders, related cognitive issues and/or substance abuse issues.

Their drug of choice is not necessarily opioids, but are related to illegal drugs such as cocaine, methamphetamine, PCP, etc., or they may have substance abuse problems related to alcohol or benzos, etc. These users may or may not have had pain when they started using illegal opioids or legal opioids obtained illegally.

They will obtain their opioid similar to those in Groups 5XA and 5XB: from diversions or illegal opioid supplies. Their path is similar, but their course to recovery and treatment is often much more difficult because it is compounded by their underlying psychiatric, mental or substance abuse-related issues. Unfortunately, mental illness is one of the many underserved categories in healthcare. Many patients will go undiagnosed for a long period, or even those who are diagnosed with mental disorder or illness may get only limited or no treatment for their conditions.

It is easy to see that someone has a problem if he or she is carried into your office with blood everywhere and broken bones sticking out of one of his or her extremities. However, it may not be easy to believe or recognize that someone who walks into your office, smiling and accompanied by a caring spouse or caregiver, may have an even greater problem.

Groups 5XD and 5XS: these are designated groups of individuals involved with opioids as dealers and suppliers. Their fate is often difficult to determine, and they will fall into any of the **Class 5** categories once they become users.

The groups and subgroups of users that I have described as "the other 60%" will almost always need a multidisciplinary approach for their treatment to be effective. One of the greatest challenges for these categories is that there are so many unknown factors, most of which are unlikely to be known prior to or during treatment. However, it goes without saying that this group will remain the greatest challenge for all of us who care about the opioid epidemic and finding meaningful solutions. Overall, **this category now accounts for more than 40% of all fatal drug overdoses in the country.**

It is also the fastest-rising group of any fatal drug-related overdose. **Drug-related deaths from other non-opioid causes account for about 34%, and drug deaths related to legal-prescription overdose account for about 26%.** Early indicators are that this 40% will continue to increase as the spread of cheap heroin, IMF and other designer/analog drugs continue to make up a significant percentage of the available illegal opioids.[3,4]

Treatments that are Available after Patients Become Addicted to Opioids

Most of the discussions so far have centered on those who do not have an opioid dependence or addiction. This is a reasonable thing to do, even though opioid addiction is also very important. The reality is that almost all patients or opioid users who died from overdose were, at some point in their initial and early stage of use, were considered "safe" before they became dependent or addicted. **Prevention and early intervention processes are significantly easier to manage than opioid addiction, thereby reducing the risks of opioid disorder progression**. Those who have an opioid dependence and/or addiction to opioids are at a higher risk of dying than those without, even though overall, there are fewer of them than are non-addicted individuals. Non-addicted patients or individuals have died and continued to die from an opioid overdose, **so it is important to know that opioid users do not have to be opioid-dependent or addicted for them to die of an overdose.**

According to a 2015 NIH publication, about two million people suffer from substance use disorder related to opioid prescriptions. Of the total number of users of opioids, it is estimated that 8% to 12% will develop an opioid use disorder.[5]

Treating Opioid Addiction

The treatment protocols mentioned throughout this book with respect to opioids and cases of opioid overdose, tolerance or dependence and/or addiction should always have naloxone available for immediate access as a life-saving drug. One of the most significant and most challenging aspects of the opioid epidemic is the treatment of opioid dependence and addiction, also called opioid use disorder.[2,6]

Over the years, dating back to the 1980s and into the early 1990s, the focus was more on enforcing the law and the criminalization of users and suppliers/dealers during the heroin epidemic. Today the focus is trending toward treatment rather than incarcerations or criminalization.[26,27]

There are several approaches that can be taken; the most practical and meaningful approach is a multidisciplinary or multimodal approach. This involves many different healthcare professionals and/or specialists/consultants. Their role will include but not limited to focusing on understanding the patients' problems, processing, and developing treatment plans that will enable meaningful recovery. The overall benefits must outweigh the risks involved in each treatment plan.

Most professionals who treat addictions and provide pain management intervention agree that the treatment of addiction is a long-term process for both the patients and the providers. The discontinuation of illegal or legal opioids does not necessarily translate to recovery. Each patient and the caregiver must fully understand that recovery requires a full and total commitment of the patient, as well as the support that the patient received prior to he or she reaching that point in the recovery process that is considered clean. Addiction, unlike tolerance or dependence, changes the neurological structure of the brain. Hence, the process of reversal/recovery will be determined in part by how much damage is done to the brain and the required restoration to normalize function to its original state.[7,8,9,10]

The Primary Medications Used to Treat
Opioid Dependence and Addicted Patients

The **Substance Abuse and Mental Health Services Administration (SAMHSA)** has established the Medication-Assisted Treatment (MAT), which uses "FDA approved medications in combination with counseling and behavioral therapies to provide a "whole patient" approach for the treatment of substance use disorder".[11]

The Narcotic Addict Treatment Act of 1974 and The Drug Addiction Treatment Act of 2000 made it possible to utilize the FDA approved medications the above medications and other services as well. However, despite the availability of these treatments, financial, psychosocial, and political obstacles (among others) make it difficult for a significant number of patients/individuals to benefit from available services. Very often, the ones that are most affected are the very poor or those who have significant psychosocial issues. They tend to need greater care but can't afford it or, because of economic or social problems, have a more significant risk of diversions of control substances.

For example, although Suboxone is available and covered by most healthcare insurance plans, the cost varies significantly from each insurance carrier, ranging from zero dollars to about $300 per prescription depending on co-pays and coinsurance payments. Without healthcare insurance, the prices are whatever the market will allow, but it is likely to be significantly higher in most cases. The other obstacle to this process is that in general, a significant number of the patients who need treatment for addictions are often the most challenging and most risky patients that any practice or medical facility will manage.

Therefore, their costs of services tend to be much greater than those of non- addicted patients. They require more frequent monitoring as well as more consultants and service-related follow-ups in order to facilitate their recovery through a multidisciplinary approach.

Another important factor is that sometimes, these addicted patients have no healthcare insurance, or they have insurance that most providers do not accept; the result is that they may not do well in treatment programs.

There are a number of reasons for this, some of which are psychosocial-related. There are times when they will need surgeries, procedures and support services that are either not covered or compensated by their healthcare insurances; or when the providers are compensated, the amount that they are paid is considered financially unsatisfactory for them to function.

Some of these patients may have significant chronic pain which will not necessarily go away with Suboxone; however, it is likely to improve their withdrawal symptoms and cravings. Therefore, these patients may go back to seeking opioids, illegal substances or whatever they considered necessary to relieve their pain, starting the cycle all over again if they are lucky to survive the potential opioid overdose.

It is important to realize that using suboxone and other similar medications in all of these structured and controlled programs does not eliminate their potential for misuse and abuse.

Primary Medications

- ➤ *Suboxone-Buprenorphine and naloxone combination*
- ➤ *Buprenorphine*
- ➤ *Methadone*
- ➤ *Naltrexone-Vivitrol*

Suboxone

This is a combination of buprenorphine (opioid partial agonist-antagonist) and naloxone (opioid antagonist). This comes in two forms: a sublingual film and sublingual tablets. **Suboxone**, **Bunavil** and **Generic Buprenorphine - Naloxone** are sublingual films. **Zubsolv** (sublingual tablet) was approved in 2013, and has the same components of buprenorphine and naloxone, with the same indication as Suboxone.

The FDA approved Suboxone and **Subutex** (sublingual tablet) in 2002 to treat opioid dependence. Subutex was discontinued in 2011.

Suboxone is one of the primary medications for patients with opioid dependence or opioid use disorder. Suboxone competes with and blocks other opioids from binding to areas in the brain called receptors. This also can help decrease pain and the amount of cravings that drive addictions associated with other opioids.

The FDA established a **Risk Evaluation and Mitigation Strategy (REMS)**, a guideline to be followed in utilizing Suboxone, with the intention of ensuring that the benefits outweigh the risks prior to starting patients on this medication. Both healthcare providers and patients are to be made aware of the medication's benefits and risks.[12,20]

Some of the advantages of Suboxone are that it is associated with less stigma compared to methadone, and it also has less potential for dependence and withdrawal. However, dependence can and will develop, as well as the potential for withdrawal, if the medication is suddenly stopped. In addition, patients can gradually be tapered off of Suboxone much easier than methadone.

Buprenorphine

Buprenorphine (opioid partial agonist-antagonist) is available in many different formulations to treat opioid dependence. It is available in the following forms:

➤ *Sublingual tablet*: **Generic Buprenorphine**
➤ *Injections:* **Sublocade**, used to treat opioid dependence; given subcutaneously approximately every month.
➤ *Sublingual tablets*: **Subutex** (discontinued in 2011).
➤ *Implant*: **Probuphine,** a buprenorphine formulation that is available in a six-month subcutaneous dose.[20]

Both buprenorphine and Suboxone are used to treat opioid dependence and addiction. Buprenorphine is sometimes used as an alternative to methadone for treating heroin addicts. It blocks other opioids as well as reduces withdrawal symptoms.[14,20,21]

Buprenorphine is also available in several formulations to treat pain:

➤ *Transdermal patch*: **Butrans Patch**, used to treat chronic pain.
➤ *Injection:* **Buprenex** – moderate to severe pain; **Generic buprenorphine** to treat moderate to severe pain.
➤ *Buccal trip*: **Belbuca** – given 1 to 2 times per day for severe chronic pain.

Methadone

Methadone is a synthetic opioid which has been around since the 1960s. It is essentially a drug consisting of two compounds in the form of isomers (I and D). This gives methadone its unique property: being able to act on receptors essentially responsible for its strong pain and addiction properties, called mu- opioid receptors. It also has an N-methyl-D-aspartate (NMDA) receptor, which is a weaker opioid receptor with less analgesic and addictive properties.[17]

Methadone has a long and variable half-life of about 24 to over 50 hours. Its half-life is much longer in opioid-tolerant patients compared to opioid-naïve patients.

When taken for opioid addiction (primarily heroin) treatment, it may remain in the body for over 36 hours from its initial dose. It is usually administered orally in pill or liquid form. In general, it is used primarily in maintenance programs to treat patients who were addicted to opioids (primarily heroin) to lessen their withdrawal symptoms without blocking other opioids. It functions as an opioid agonist without the significant euphoria, sedation or cravings associated with other more addictive opioids by blocking or reducing these effects. Methadone maintenance treatment programs also focus on enhancing medical, behavioral as well as psychosocial issues.[16]

Methadone is also used in the treatment of moderate to severe chronic pain; most often, oral formulation is used. It is prescribed about two to three times per day for pain management and once a day for opioid use disorder and methadone treatment programs. Pain relief from methadone dosing is expected to last about four to eight hours. There are, however, SC/IM/IV (given by skin, muscle or vain); these formulations, although available, are rarely used for administration. When using in the non-oral form, it is used for acute conditions, but they are much better and safer alternatives. One of the challenges of using oral methadone for chronic pain is that its analgesic effect may take up to three to five days before the patients feel that they're getting any benefit, even if the medication is still present at a very high level in their system. In addition, methadone is associated with cardiac arrhythmia, the abnormal conduction of electrical impulse in the heart (prolonged QT), and as indicated above, a very long half-life.

The patients can and often overdose partly because they're taking more medications than prescribed, hoping for faster pain relief. It is therefore imperative and critical when starting patients on oral methadone to ensure that detailed patient education with demonstrated understanding is done to reduce the risks of overdose from methadone, particularly within the early phases of treatment. Also, a low starting dose is required taking into consideration the patients' age, comorbidities, and other factors.

When appropriately used, methadone is still relatively safe compared to other opioids such as IMF, heroin, or even some prescription opioids. The death rate from methadone, although significant, has remained relatively low compared to the other opioids mentioned; see the graph below.[18]

Overdose Deaths Involving Opioids, by Type of Opioid, United States, 2000-2016

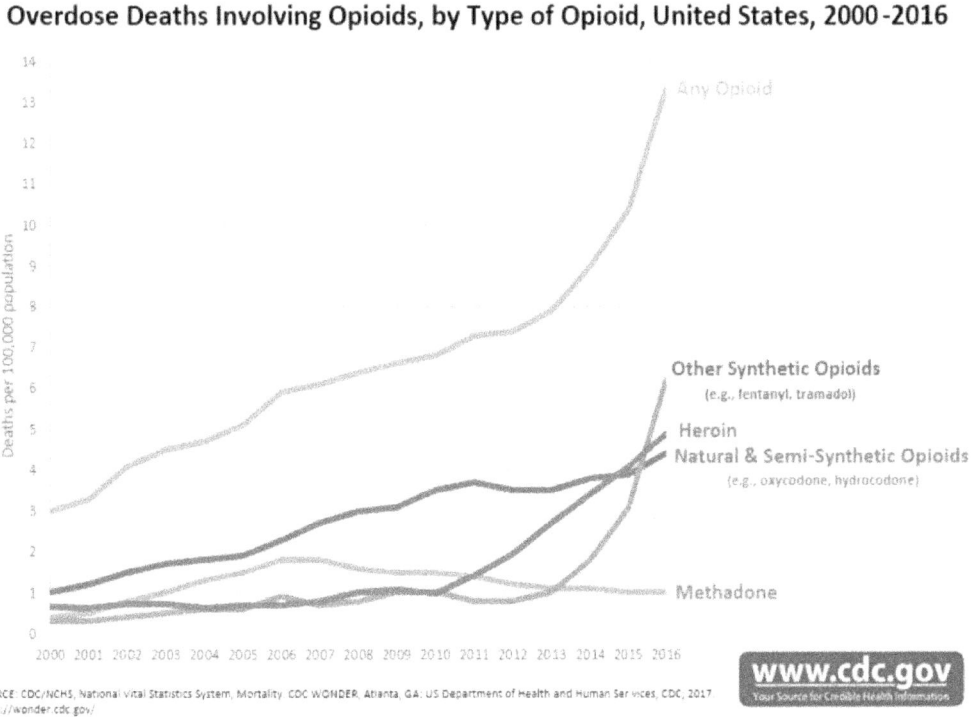

SOURCE: CDC/NCHS, National Vital Statistics System, Mortality. CDC WONDER, Atlanta, GA: US Department of Health and Human Services, CDC; 2017. https://wonder.cdc.gov/

It is important to note that methadone is highly addictive, and if it is suddenly stopped, it will lead to severe withdrawal. It is much more regulated than Suboxone. Unfortunately, methadone patients sometimes use illicit or illegally manufactured opioids as well as legal opioids to help control their pain or to gain additional euphoria.

However, if under strict supervision, patients can tolerate significantly higher dosages, resulting in better pain control as their level of tolerance increase. The cost of methadone is generally less than that of Suboxone.[13,14,15]

Naltrexone

Naltrexone is an opioid antagonist which works by blocking other opioids, significantly decreasing the cravings often associated with withdrawal. It can be taken as a pill or as an injection for opioid addiction.

It may also be taken in a pill or liquid form, placed under the tongue for treatment of chronic pain in dosages that are considered **low-dose naltrexone** or **ultra-low-dose naltrexone**. The mechanism of action is dose-dependent and different for standard naltrexone compared with a low-dose and ultra-low-dose naltrexone. Naltrexone is a non-addictive opioid.

Naltrexone Pill

Naltrexone pill formulation may be administered orally once a day, and also treats opioid dependence. Patients also are required to be at least seven to ten days opioid- free. This medication in both forms can also be used to treat alcohol dependence.[18]

Vivitrol

Naltrexone, in its injectable form, is called **Vivitrol**. It can be used to treat opioid dependence. Vivitrol is administered by injecting it into the muscle once every four weeks. The patients must be opioid-free for about seven to ten days, that is, have not taken opioids for that duration. This significantly helps in preventing relapse following opioid detoxification. This may be ideal for addicts who are opioid- dependent and have been deprived of opioids; for example, due to hospitalization, incarceration or others.[19]

The Epocrates medical prescription database lists the price of naltrexone 50 mg (30 tablets) at $43.09; while Vivitrol 380 mg/vial (one carton, one vial) in its injectable form is at $1,539.00, one single-dose/month. So, there is a choice! However, bear in mind that the cost of the medications is often determined by your healthcare insurance plan and many other factors. The standard dose for naltrexone is 50 mg daily (most common use), 100 mg every other day, or 150 mg every three days.

Low-Dose and Ultra-Low-Dose Naltrexone

Low-dose naltrexone, defined as 1.5 - 4.5 mg once daily, has been used to treat many chronic pain conditions with success. The medications can be taken by pill form or from concentrated liquid form placed under the tongue. The effect is believed to be related to anti-inflammatory, analgesic as well as possible immune-mediated factors. Studies have shown that patients do get decreased pain response from chronic pain related to fibromyalgia, Crohn's disease, irritable bowel syndrome, and autoimmune conditions, among others.[22,23]

Ultra-low-dose naltrexone, defined as less than 0.1 mg dose, is also being studied and believed to have an analgesic effect with a mechanism involving the endogenous opioids.[24,25]

Other medications

Clonidine, although not commonly used as the others that are listed, is used to help reduce some withdrawal symptoms associated with opioid dependence and addiction. It is also commonly used for hypertension treatment.

References, Recommended Readings and Resources

1. Levy B, Paulozzi L, Mack KA, Jones CM. Trends in Opioid Analgesic-Prescribing Rates by Specialty, U.S., 2007-2012. Am J Prev Med. 2015 Sep;49(3):409-13.Apr 18, 2015.Opioid Overdose Prescribing Data. https://www.ncbi.nlm.nih.gov/pmc/articles/PMC6034509/ Accessed May 26, 2018.

2. Effective Medical Treatment of Opiate Addiction. National Institutes of Health. Consensus Development Conference Statement. November 17-19, 1997. https://consensus.nih.gov/1997/1998treatopiateaddiction108html.htm Accessed June30, 2018.

3. The Centers for Disease Control and Prevention. Understanding the Epidemic. https://www.cdc.gov/drugoverdose/epidemic/index.html. Last visited June 16, 2018.

4. Puja Seth, Ph.D.; Lawrence Scholl, Ph.D.; Rose A. Rudd, MSPH; Sarah Bacon, Ph.D., *MMMWR*. Overdose deaths involving opioids, cocaine, and psychostimulants – the United States, 2015 – 2016. https://www.cdc.gov/ mmwr/volumes/67/wr/mm6712a1.htm.Accessed May 5, 2018.

5. NIH. National Institute on Drug Abuse. Opioid overdose crisis.https:// www.drugabuse.gov/drugs-abuse/opioids/opioid-overdose-crisis.Accessed June 4, 2018.

6. Gary Peltz, MD, Ph.D.; Thomas C. Südhof, MD. The Neurobiology of Opioid Addiction and the Potential for Prevention Strategies. *JAMA*. 2018;319(20):2071-2072. May 22/29, 2018 https://jamanetwork.com/journals/jama/issue/319/20 . Accessed June 30,2018.

7. National Institute on Drug Abuse. Principles of Drug Addiction Treatment: A Research-Based Guide. Third edition. Last reviewed December 2012. https://www.drugabuse.gov/sites/default/files/podat_1.pdf. Accessed July 2, 2018.

8. Thomas Kosten, Tony P George. The Neurobiology of Opioid Dependence: Implications for Treatment. NIH. Science & Practice Perspectives. 13-20. August 2002. https://www.ncbi.nlm.nih.gov/pubmed/18567959 Accessed July 7, 2018.

9. George F. Koob. The neurobiology of addiction: a neuroadaptational view relevant for diagnosis.08 August 2006. https://onlinelibrary.wiley.com/doi/abs/10.1111/j.1360-0443.2006.01586.x Last accessed June 30, 2018

10. George F Koob Ph.D., Nora D Volkow MD. Neurobiology of addiction: a neurocircuitry analysis. The Lancet Psychiatry Volume 3, Issue 8, August 2016, Pages 760-773 https://www.sciencedirect.com/science/article/pii/S2215036616001048 Last accessed on June 30, 2018.

11. Substance Abuse and Mental Health Services Administration. Programs & Campaigns » Medication-Assisted Treatment » Medication and Counseling Treatment » Methadone. https://www.samhsa.gov/medication-assisted-treatment/treatment/methadone Last accessed June 30, 2018.

12. Risk Evaluation and Mitigation Strategy (REMS). Reckitt Benckiser Pharmaceuticals Inc. SUBOXONE® (buprenorphine and naloxone) sublingual tablet CIII Buprenorphine (opioid partial agonist-antagonist) Naloxone (opioid antagonist). Dec. 2011https://www.fda.gov/downloads/Drugs/DrugSafety/PostmarketDrugSafetyInformationforPatientsandProviders/UCM285895.pdf Last accessed June 30, 2018.

13. Substance Abuse and Mental Health Services Administration. Programs & Campaigns » Medication-Assisted Treatment » Medication and Counseling Treatment » Suboxone. https://www.samhsa.gov/medication-assisted-treatment/treatment/Suboxone Last accessed June 30, 2018

14. Substance Abuse and Mental Health Services Administration. Programs & Campaigns » Medication-Assisted Treatment » Medication and Counseling Treatment » Buprenorphine. https://www.samhsa.gov/medication-assisted-treatment/treatment/buprenorphine Last accessed June 30, 2018.

15. Substance Abuse and Mental Health Services Administration. Programs & Campaigns » Medication-Assisted Treatment » Medication and Counseling Treatment » methadone. https://www.samhsa.gov/medication-assisted-treatment/treatment/methadone Last accessed June 30, 2018.

16. Eliseo Salinas, MD, MSc. Relmada Therapeutics. d-Methadone: A Novel Approach for Neuropathic Pain. 03/12/2015. https://www.dddmag.com/article/2015/03/d-methadone-novel-approach-neuropathic-pain Last accessed June 30, 2018.

17. Center for Disease Control and Prevention CDC. Opioid Data Analysis. https://www.cdc.gov/drugoverdose/data/analysis.html Last accessed July 1, 2018.

18. Substance Abuse and Mental Health Services Administration. Programs & Campaigns » Medication-Assisted Treatment » Medication and Counseling Treatment » Naltrexone. https://www.samhsa.gov/medication-assisted-treatment/treatment/naltrexone Last accessed June 30, 2018.

19. U.S. Food and Drug Administration. (2016). FDA Approves First Buprenorphine Implant for Treatment of Opioid Dependence. May 26, 2016. https://www.fda.gov/NewsEvents/Newsroom/PressAnnouncements/ucm503719.htm Last accessed July 2, 2018

20. Center for Substance Abuse Treatment. Clinical Guidelines for the Use of Buprenorphine in the Treatment of Opioid Addiction. Treatment Improvement Protocol (TIP) Series 40. DHHS Publication No. (SMA) 04-3939. Rockville, Md: Substance Abuse and Mental Health Services Administration, 2004,https://www.naabt.org/documents/TIP40.pdf Last accessed July 2, 2018.

21. Jarred Younger, Luke Parkitny, and David McLain. The use of low-dose naltrexone (LDN) as a novel anti-inflammatory treatment for chronic pain. Clin Rheumatol. 2014; 33(4): 451–459. February 15, 2014. https://www.ncbi.nlm.nih.gov/pmc/articles/PMC3962576/ Last accessed July 29, 2018.

22. Miriam E. Tucker. Low-dose Naltrexone Explored as Option for Chronic Pain. March 16, 2018. https://www.medscape.com/viewarticle/894020 Last accessed July 29, 2018.

23. Lindsay H. Burns. Pain Therapeutics, Inc. Ultra-low-dose opioid antagonists enhance opioid analgesia while reducing tolerance, dependence and addictive properties. 2005.http://paintrials.com/publications/Capasso8.pdf Last accessed July 29, 2018.

24. Ultra-Low Dose Naltrexone – For Lower Opiate Tolerance – Research Summary. November 4, 2015.https://www.khemcorp.com/ultra-low-dose-naltrexone-for-lower-opiate-tolerance-research-summary/ Last accessed July 29, 2018.
25. Rebecca Tiger. Race, Class, and the Framing of Drug Epidemics. December 18, 2017. https://contexts.org/articles/race-class-drugs/ Last accessed July 29, 2018.
26. Race and the Drug War. http://www.drugpolicy.org/issues/race-and-drug-war

    Last accessed July 29, 2018.

Chapter 10

Some of the Programs that are Available for Opioid Dependence and Opioid Use Disorder Patients

The illegal use of drugs by different routes, particular intravenously, has been around for generations. Some of the challenges that come with this is trying to balance the need for law enforcement or crime prevention versus healthcare needs, saving lives, and the reduction and prevention of diseases. Most of us have some knowledge of HIV/AIDS infection, hepatitis and other infections causing significant mortality compounded by IV drug abuse such as the use of heroin.

This problem is not unique to one community, state or country; rather, it affects many globally. As a result of this, many countries have tried to find ways to deal with the various challenges that come with drug abuse and addictions. Some of these methods or actions are controversial, to say the least, while others have gained support on both sides of the issues. Because of the long history associated with some of these methods, there are at least some statistical data to help better evaluate their risks and benefits.

Supervised Injection Sites

Supervised injection sites are also called **safe injection sites**, **supervised consumption facilities**, or **sanitary consumption facilities**.[1] They function as healthcare facilities or clinics where addicts or intravenous drug users can go and inject themselves, usually with their illegally owned drugs, more safely.

They will do this under the supervision of trained medical and nonmedical personnel, and they are generally able to administer life-saving measures including drugs such as naloxone. They will also provide counseling as well as referrals to other services or healthcare providers that may be of benefit to the abusers.

Other services may include referrals or counseling regarding drug rehab for addicts, wound-care treatments or pregnancy testing.[1] There are reported to be over 120 of these facilities throughout the world, with the largest and most well known in North America. It is called **Insite**, located in Vancouver, British Columbia, Canada. They are present in other countries such as Australia, Switzerland, Germany, Denmark, and the Netherlands, to name a few.[2,3] Most of these were established long before there was an opioid epidemic in the United States. Some of them came about when HIV/AIDS and heroin were of significant concern for many countries. Now, the concern in this country is the opioid epidemic related to drug-overdose deaths which keep increasing. Drug users primarily consume their opioids by intravenous route, and sharing of needles is very common. The previous concern was controlling the spread of infection, and hence, the spread of diseases such as HIV/AIDS and hepatitis. Today, infection is still a concern, but of more significant interest are the ever-escalating deaths from opioid overdoses via IV drug use.[4]

Switzerland established its **Heroin-Assisted Treatment (HAT)** program in 1994, which was successful in reducing and regulating heroin use and abuse, as well as decreasing the spread of infection such as HIV/AIDS and deaths. Other countries have adopted similar models. This program is a supervised drug injection program similar to those in North America. The HAT program provided patients with **prescription-grade heroin**.[2,3] Insite was established in 2003. Since it opened, it has served thousands of drug users and has reported saving many lives. It is also being associated with the decreased cost to the city of Vancouver related to healthcare and drug overdoses.[5]

In September 2011, the Supreme Court of Canada voted unanimously (9 to 0) to keep Insite open amid lawsuits and challenges intended to close it. Part of the conclusion from the Canadian Supreme Court's decision is, as written by Chief Justice Beverley McLachlin:[6,7]

"Insite saves lives. Its benefits have been proven. There has been no discernible negative impact on public safety and health objectives of Canada during its eight years of operation."

Since Insite opened in 2003, more than 3.6 million users have been supervised while injecting drugs; more than 6,440 overdoses interventions without deaths have occurred.

There also have been more than 50,000 treatments administered for clinic visits, for example, to treat wounds and perform pregnancy testing.

In Canada and a significant number of countries in Europe, many studies have shown that facilities like Insite have been successful in saving lives and preventing the spread of infections. Also, an associated reduction in healthcare costs, as well as crime associated with drug use and abuse, have been recorded. Because of the success of Insite, Canada now has more than 20 new sites similar to it since 2015.[6,7]

What Can We Learn from Canada and the Rest of the World?

Canada has a population of about 37 million people; we have a population of approximately 328 million people.[18] The United States and Canada are first and second in the world with respect to the use of opioids.[17] For 2017, Canada reported about 4,000 deaths related to opioid overdoses, and we have projected about 49,000. The percentage of death associated with fentanyl or IMF in Canada is about 72%; in the United States, it is probably safe to say that ours is perhaps in the neighborhood of about 55% to 60%, considering about 60% of all opioid deaths are via non- prescription or illegal drugs including fentanyl and its analogs, which is projected to be at about 30,000 deaths in 2017.[15,16]

By looking at the numbers and further reading, one can clearly see that Canada definitely has an escalating opioid crisis that doesn't appear to be at the level of an opioid epidemic (of course, each country will determine what their epidemic is, or when they have one). In theory, if all things were equal in Canada, and if it has the same population as the United States, we would expect about 20% to 30% fewer people dying from opioids in Canada. This number has the potential for significant variability depending on other non-opioid drug- related deaths as well as several other factors.

Of note in 2016, approximately 55% of the deaths from opioid overdose in Canada was related to fentanyl or its analogs; this is apparently around where we were in 2017. Therefore, things can change really quickly.[16,22]

Canada and so many other countries have taken some very aggressive and (sometimes) controversial approaches to their drug problems. Some of these are discussed in this chapter.

In addition to supervised injection sites, Canada has also started or enacted:

➢ Program for prescription-grade heroin to treat addiction – this is also part of some treatment protocols in countries like Switzerland and Germany.[23,24]

➢ Dispensing program for addicts to obtain opioids (Dilaudid/ hydromorphone) from vending machines.[25,26]

➢ National legalization of marijuana. Many believe that marijuana or components of it may be very effective in treating pain or addiction- related symptoms.[27,28]

It should be pointed out that although these treatments and options are available in Canada, a review of some of the other available treatment options found them to be as extensive, thorough and productive as those we have here in the United States or other countries. However, the ones listed here are often among those that are more frequently discussed, probably because of the controversies surrounding them.[13]

Just like Insite and related centers, these programs are not without controversies and have significant opposition from many quarters. We spoke about the Supreme Court decision in Canada to keep Insite and facilities like them open and functioning in a similar manner. However, there is still opposition to these sites and to other programs considered by some as more of an encouragement to drug addicts and abusers rather than solutions to the opioid crisis. The new (June 2018) administration of Doug Ford in Ontario has been in the news recently for its apparent stand against facilities like Insite, even though the Canadian Supreme Court voted unanimously to keep them open.[19,20,21] So how will we handle our opioid epidemic with the information and knowledge that we have gained from facilities and actions taken in Canada and around the world? [13]

What are We Doing in the United States
Concerning These Facilities and Programs?

In the United States, there is currently no clinic that directly functions the way Insite or other supervised clinics do. There are clinics, associations and non-profit organizations that offer some of the services provided by supervised clinics.

These services range from clean needle exchange, social service intervention, referrals to educational services, detoxification or drug rehabilitation programs for addiction, and support groups, among others. Their state laws do not necessarily sanction these facilities' operations.

Some states have enacted laws that allow or sanction **harm reduction organizations** to operate without individuals associated with the organizations subjected to prosecution or as part of criminal charges. These are organizations that will provide services such as syringe/needle exchange, education, and others to at-risk groups of individuals. This is intended to reduce the potential spread of infectious diseases (such as hepatitis and HIV), overdoses and deaths.[14]

In the United States, it is illegal to administer intravenous drugs, both at the state and federal level – unless of course, you are a healthcare provider or in a healthcare facility and usually under a doctor's supervision. This applies to legal drugs.

No one is, of course allowed to administer illicit drugs or to operate any establishment that facilitates the use of illegal drugs.

San Francisco in California had planned to open two supervised clinics in July 2018; we are now approaching the end of the year 2018. The clinics are expected to function similar to models established in Vancouver. These facilities are expected to save approximately $3.5 million per year in medical costs usually incurred by overdoses. Because of state and federal regulations prohibiting the functioning of such clinics, San Francisco is hoping to have these facilities funded privately.[8]

As of September 2018, there is still a very strong opposition at the federal and local levels regarding the opening of safe injection sites. A prototype of the clinics has been "opened" but are not functioning in the way they are intended to operate. This is primarily the result of both federal and local opposition and the associated legal hurdles that must be overcome.[31,32,33,34]

Plans are also in progress for clinics in Philadelphia, Seattle, and Baltimore and other places to be established and function similar to Insite. However, all these clinics or facilities will have legal, political, social and humanitarian hurdles to overcome before any of them can open and function without the fear of employees, volunteers or drug users being arrested and charged at these facilities.[9]

On September 5, 2018, the American Society of Addiction Medicine (ASAM)'s *ASAM Weekly* publication brought our attention to an op-ed in the *New York Times* on August 27, 2018, by Deputy Attorney General Rod J. Rosenstein, titled "Fight Drug Abuse, Don't Subsidize It."

In this article, Mr. Rosenstein clearly expressed his strong opposition to safe injection sites in the United States as a treatment option that would help reduce the impact of the opioid epidemic.

He explained in this article his reasons for his opposition. He also reminded us that it is a federal felony to maintain any facility for the use of illegal drugs. Punishment may include up to 20 years in prison, fines, and forfeitures of the property involved in the crime. The Department of Justice is expected to take aggressive action against any such sites and/or its operators for being involved in criminal activities. It is reasonable to assume that this is the official position of the federal government. Therefore, all states and/or cities, including California, Seattle, Massachusetts, Colorado, Philadelphia, and others, that are planning or exploring establishing safe injection sites are now put on notice.[36]

As the opioid epidemic continues to be a significant factor in the United States, politicians/lawmakers, as well as citizens, will have to make decisions in terms of what they think is best for their states and the country as a whole.

Other Programs

In Vermont, there is a **pre-charge program**. This basically entails providing the options of jail versus treatment for offenders with minor offenses that are related to drugs and addiction.

These individuals are assigned a counselor responsible for their supervision or facilitation of possible employment, housing, drug treatment program, and others. The individual is also expected to participate in community service related to the crime they committed. If these individuals successfully complete the program, they will avoid being charged and possibly sentenced for their crime.[29]

Detoxification (Detox) is the removal of toxins from the body. Toxins result from the breakdown of substances such as drugs, natural herbs or even food that we ingest. The drugs may be legal or illegal drugs. Although the body has its own mechanisms or ways of getting rid of toxins, sometimes there's so much accumulation that additional means are required to help the process. Detoxification is a means of restoring the body to its neutral non-opioid or non-drug state. This requires the control and management of sometimes mild to unbearable withdrawal symptoms, which are generally a necessary pathway to detox.

The level of the detox the users must go through depends on many factors, including the extent of their drug tolerance, dependence or addiction. These factors often correlate to potential withdrawal symptoms, which helps to determine the appropriate level of detox.

Detox is the best approach from a multidisciplinary framework. The option of inpatient versus outpatient detox often depends on the potential withdrawal symptoms, extent of addiction status, family structures, finances, and sometimes patients' preferences, among others.

Medical detox or Medical-model detox will involve an interdisciplinary medical team such as physicians – these may include primary addiction and/or substance abuse specialists, psychiatrists, other consultants, nurses, psychologists, social workers, etc.

Among the functions served are the appropriate maintenance and management of physical and psychological withdrawal symptoms and cravings. This will be achieved by the interdisciplinary team's applications specific to their discipline as well as medications management.[10,11]

In May 2018, the US FDA approved **Lucemyra (lofexidine hydrochloride)**, the first medication indicated specifically for the treatment of withdrawal symptoms associated with the abrupt discontinuation of opioids in adults. The medication is expected to decrease the severity of withdrawal symptoms (it may not prevent them), and the duration of treatment for each case is 14 days. Although the medication itself is not used for the treatment of opioid use disorder in the United States, it may be incorporated in both outpatient and inpatient detox programs.

In the United Kingdom, it is sold as **BritLofex** and is used in their detoxification programs for opioid addicts.[30,35]

An **Inpatient detox program** may last for seven to 10 days or even 30 days, and longer on occasion. One of the primary reasons for detox is to control withdrawal symptoms and pronounced cravings, hence decreasing the risk of relapse. During the time of detox, depending on the level of severity of withdrawal symptoms and craving for drugs, the drug users may revert to using the drugs for which they are being detoxed from (**relapse**). This occurs particularly if they do not have a good support structure, or if they are treated by outpatient centers where there is better access to available drugs.

One of the risks involved with **relapse** is that sometimes, some of these patients although going through withdrawal after discharge and having had no significant opioids for a period, are now considered to be in opioid-naïve states. This makes them very susceptible to overdose and death upon re-entry to drug use.

There are so many cases wherein individuals had completed detoxification or drug rehab and died soon after from drug overdose when they go back to consuming the same quantity of drugs that they used before detoxing.

Because of the loss of tolerance during their abstinence from drugs, their risk of overdosing is significantly increased. Their body is no longer able to tolerate the large amounts of drugs they were accustomed to before. Hence, they now become easier victims of drug overdose.

Outpatient detox programs often take a similar approach to inpatient programs. However, the patients who are treated are expected to experience far fewer withdrawal symptoms than inpatients. Usually, their social and financial structures are much better. Their risks of relapsing are still significant, but with appropriate support and a multidisciplinary approach, outpatient treatment is still a viable option.

Regardless of how good and effective the detox program one may have completed is, the greatest challenge lies ahead. Patients are now expected to continue and sustain a maintenance program. Again, the multidisciplinary approach is critical, as well as a support group and family structure for a long- term and more lasting recovery.[11,12]

Some Commonly Used Behavioral Therapies

These supporting therapies (among others) are used both in inpatient and outpatient settings:[11]

1. ***Family therapy***: This essentially incorporates the family into the care and well-being of patients in order to educate them and facilitates direct involvement during therapy to enhance recovery.

2. ***Cognitive behavioral therapy***: This is the principle of therapy wherein it is believed that our feelings and behavior work in conjunction to support substance abuse; therefore, modifying them will modify substance abuse.

3. ***Motivational interviewing***: It is a collaborative style of counseling which invokes the patient's motivation for and commitment to change.

4. ***Contingency management***: This provides rewards for drug-free status, and counteracts rewards by continued use of the substance.

Relapse – What to Do?

The path to recovery or sobriety, or being drug-free again is attainable, but it is not easy. For most people who are trying to put their lives back together and become drug-free essentially, the challenges are always there. It is best to consider exiting a detox program when the user is without drugs for the duration of that program; consider that time a **period of pause**.

It is an essential part of the recovery process, but **it is not the recovery itself.**

The greatest and most challenging time lies ahead for the user.

Relapses are often driven by cravings for drugs, accessibility to drugs, lack of support, and the user's desire for drugs, among other things. The people who care about their loved ones and are involved in their lives must realize the importance of structural support from family and close friends. This support at the end of detox is as essential as it was in the initial phase of therapy. Following up with multidisciplinary team members is of critical importance to continue the recovery process. This must be done consistently, even when things appear to be going well.[11,12]

References, Recommended Readings and Resources

1. Supervised injection sites. http://www.vch.ca/public-health/harm-reduction/supervised-consumption-sites. Accessed March 20,2018.
2. Heroin-assisted treatment in Switzerland: successfully regulating the sup-ply and use of a high-risk injectable drug. *Submitted by: Transform. 10th Jan 2017.* https://www.tdpf.org.uk/blog/heroin-assisted-treatment-swit-zerland-successfully-regulating-supply-and-use-high-risk-0.Accessed March 21, 2018.
3. Ella Müller-Baum. Switzerland to Get New SupervisedInjection Facility in 2017. June 22, 2016. https://www.talkingdrugs.org/ switzerland-new-supervised-injection-facility-in-2017.Accessed March 21, 2018.
4. Erin Schumaker. To Fight the Opioid Crisis, Health Experts Recommend Safe Places to Shoot Up. HuffPost. 10/31/2017. https:// www.huffing- tonpost.com/entry/safe-drug-injection-sites-research_us_59f75a4ae- 4b0aec146793968. Accessed March 21, 2018.

5. Ashifa Kassam. Canada offers places for addicts to shoot up safely. Can the US copy the model? June 23, 2017. https://www.theguardian. com/us-news/2017/jun/23/vancouver-supervised-injection-clinic- heroin.Accessed June 20, 2018

6. Kirk Makin, Sunny Dhillon, and Ingrid Peritz, Supreme Court ruling open doors to drug injection clinics across Canada. September 30, 2011. https:// www.theglobeandmail.com/news/british-columbia/ supreme-court- ruling- opens-doors-to-drug-injection-clinics-across-canada/article4182250/. Accessed June 26, 2018.

7. Mike Blanchfield, Supreme Court OKs Insite Safe Injection Site in Unanimous Ruling. 09/30/2011. https://www.huffingtonpost. ca/2011/09/30/su- preme-court-insite-unanimous-ruling_n_988733. html. Accessed June 26, 2018.

8. Mark Lieber, CNN. Safe injection sites in San Francisco could be first in the US. February 7, 2018, https://www.cnn.com/2018/02/07/health/ safe-injec- tion- sites-San-Francisco-opioid-epidemic-bn/index.html. Accessed March 2018.

9. Jericka Duncan Philadelphia considers opening site for heroin users to shoot up safely. Accessed June 26, 2018.

10. Substance Abuse and Mental Health Services Administration Detoxification and Substance Abuse Treatment. Last revised 2015. https://store.samhsa. gov/shin/content/SMA15-4131/SMA15-4131.pdf. Accessed July 2, 2018.

11. National Institute on Drug Abuse. Principles of Drug Addiction Treatment: A Research-Based Guide. Third edition. Last reviewed December 2012. https://www.drugabuse.gov/sites/default/files/ podat_1.pdf. Accessed July 2, 2018

12. Thomas Kosten, Tony P George. The Neurobiology of Opioid Dependence:Implications for Treatment. NIH. Science & Practice Perspectives. 13-20 August 2002. https://www.researchgate.net/ publication/5288549_The_ Neurobiology_of_Opioid_Dependence_ Implications_for_Treatment. Accessed July 7, 2018.

13. Get the facts on the opioid crisis in Canada. https://www.canada.ca/en/ services/health/campaigns/drug-prevention.html. Accessed August 19, 2018.

14. Harm Reduction Coalition. http://harmreduction.org/. Last visited August 17, 2018.

15. NIH. National Institute of Drug Abuse. Overdose Death Rates Revised August 2018. https://www.drugabuse.gov/related-topics/trends- statistics/ overdose- death-rates. Accessed August 16, 2018.

16. National report: Apparent opioid-related deaths in Canada. (released June 2018). https://www.canada.ca/en/public-health/services/ publications/healthy-living/national-report-apparent-opioid-related- deaths- re- leased-june-2018.html. Last visited August 19, 2018.

17. Keith Humphreys. Americans use far more opioids than anyone else in the world. March 5, 2017. https://www.washingtonpost.com/news/ wonk/ wp/2017/03/15/americans-use-far-more-opioids-than-anyone- else-in- the-world/?utm_term=.be634a22752e. Accessed August 19, 2018.

18. The U.S. and World Population Clock.https://www.census.gov/ popclock/. Last visited August 19, 2018.

19. The Canadian Press. Ontario Health Minister Christine Elliott puts3 over- dose prevention sites on hold. Province holding off opening 3 overdose-prevention sites intended to help fight the opioid crisis. Aug 13, 2018. https://www.cbc.ca/news/canada/toronto/ontario-holding-off-overdose-preven- tion-sites-1.4783592. Last visited August 19, 2018.

20. Ryan Maloney. Doug Ford Digs In Against Safe Injection Sites At 1st De- bate. May 7, 2018. https://www.huffingtonpost.ca/2018/05/07/ doug-ford- safe- injection-sites-debate_a_23429304/. Last visited August 19, 2018.

21. Kieran Delamont. What could the PC government's review of supervised injection sites mean in Ottawa? July 26, 2018. https:// ottawacitizen.com/ news/local-news/what-could-the-pc-governments- review- of-super- vised-injection-sites-mean-in-ottawa. Last visited August 19, 2018.

22. Brian Hutchinson. Canada's first safe injection site struggles with the rise of fentanyl. September 1, 2017. https://www.macleans.ca/news/canada/cana- das- first-safe-injection-site-struggles-with-the-rise-of-fentanyl/. Last visit- ed August 19, 2018.

23. The Canadian Press. Canada now allows prescription heroin in severe opioid addiction. Sep 08, 2016. http://www.cbc.ca/news/canada/ british- co- lumbia/canada-now-allows-prescription-heroin-in-severe-opioid-addiction-1.3753312. Accessed August 19, 2018.

24. Kyle Duggan. Health Canada speeding up access to prescription heroin, methadone. Mar 26, 2018. https://ipolitics.ca/2018/03/26/ health-canada- speeding-up-access-to-prescription-heroin-methadone/. Accessed August 19, 2018.

25. Digital Reporter CKNW. Opioid vending machines among 'out of the box' overdose solutions at Vancouver forum. June 7, 2018. https:// globalnews. ca/news/4261182/opioid-vending-machines-vancouver/. Accessed August 19, 2018.

26. Amanda Coletta. Canada's fix to the opioid crisis: Vending machines that distribute prescription opioids to addicts. January 24, 2018. https://www. washingtonpost.com/news/worldviews/wp/2018/01/24/ the- canadian-fix- to-the-opioid-crisis-a-vending-machine-that- distributes- prescription-opi- oids-to-addicts/?utm_term=.fe099b6d3692. Accessed August 19, 2018.

27. Monique Scotti. National Online Journalist, Politics Global News Marijuana legalization Bill C-45 officially passes Senate vote, heading for royal as- sent. June 19, 2018. https://globalnews.ca/news/4282677/ pot-bill-senate- passes/. Accessed June 20, 2018.

28. Peter Zimonjic. CBC News. Senate passes pot bill, paving the way for le- gal cannabis in 8 to 12 weeks. June 19, 2018. https://www.cbc.ca/ news/ politics/senate-passes-government-pot-bill-1.4713222. Accessed June 20, 2018.

29. Innovative Criminal Justice Programs in Vermont. http://forms.vermont-law.edu/criminaljustice/PreCharge.cfm. Accessed August 19, 2018.

30. The U.S. Food and Drug Administration. FDA approves the first non- opioid treatment for management of opioid withdrawal symptoms in adults. May 16, 2018. https://www.fda.gov/newsevents/newsroom/pressannouncements/ucm607884.htm. Accessed September 22, 2018.

31. Sarah Holder. A Controversial Fix for Overdose Deaths: Safe Injection Sites. September 5, 2018. https://www.citylab.com/equity/2018/09/building-a- safe- space-for-san-franciscos-addicts/568942/. Accessed September 22, 2018.

32. Victoria Colliver, Dan Goldberg and Rachel Roubein. Trump administration warns California against 'safe' opioid injection sites. 08/28/2018. https://www.politico.com/story/2018/08/28/san-franciscos-safe-injection-sites-justice-department-759017. Accessed September 22, 2018.

33. Joe Khalil. Legal Injection Sites Could Soon Come to California, but Not Everyone is On Board. September 3, 2018. https://fox40. com/2018/09/03/ legal- injection-sites-could-soon-come-to-california- but-not-everyone-is- on-board/. Accessed September 22, 2018.

34. Sam Brock. San Francisco Preparing to Open Safe Injection Sites. August 17, 2018. https://www.nbcbayarea.com/news/local/San- Francisco- Preparing-to-Open-Safe-Injection-Sites-491151661.html. Accessed September 22, 2018.

35. New Treatments for Opiate Addiction to Consider for 2017 (Updated for 2018). https://family-intervention.com/blog/new-treatments-for- opiate- addiction-to-consider-for-2017/. Accessed September 22, 2018.

36. Rod J. Rosenstein. Fight Drug Abuse, Don't Subsidize It. Aug. 27, 2018. https://www.nytimes.com/2018/08/27/opinion/opioids-heroin- injection- sites.html. Accessed October 2, 2018.

Chapter 11

Naloxone: A Life-Saving Drug for Opioid Overdose

What is Naloxone?

Naloxone is the drug of choice for saving lives that are in jeopardy due to opioid overdose. This drug is effective only for opioid overdose, at reportedly greater than 90% effective. However, it may or may not be effective on illegally manufactured opioids or synthetic opioid analogs. Regardless, it is still recommended to be used in all opioids or suspected opioids and unknown-drug overdose. As mentioned earlier, opioids cause death primarily by shutting down the area in the brain responsible for breathing and respiration.

Everyone who hopes to be helpful and useful in the fight against the opioid epidemic needs to and must understand the importance of naloxone in saving lives.

Naloxone is an opioid antagonist which acts by reversing the effects of opioids on the central nervous system (it does so by displacing opioids from their receptors). This generally results in the overdose being removed or significantly reduced, and the body returning close to its normal state of function before the overdose. Once revived, the recipient of naloxone is likely to experience withdrawal from opioids (see some symptoms below).

Opioid Overdose Symptoms

- ➢ Difficulty in arising or staying awake (lethargy or somnolence)
- ➢ Slow, shallow breathing or no breathing
- ➢ Unable to keep the body upright (limp)
- ➢ Small or pinpoint pupils
- ➢ Loss or decreased level of consciousness
- ➢ Loss of pulse or slow heart rate
- ➢ Cold and clammy hands
- ➢ Pale complexion and blue lips.

Opioids Withdrawal Symptoms

Opioid withdrawal is a physiological response to decreased levels or absence of opioids in the body. This occurs because of changes in the levels of compounds called neurotransmitters, primarily dopamine and noradrenaline. Dopamine is usually responsible for the pleasure and euphoria experience with opioids, and noradrenaline is responsible for increased energy and alertness. Noradrenaline is generally suppressed by dopamine. It is the adjustments and readjustments of different levels of these neurotransmitters and the associated neurotransmitters that lead to opioid withdrawal. Neurotransmitters modify each other and work in concert with other neurotransmitters. In addition, different drugs may have varied and different effects on different neurotransmitters.

Most patients who will demonstrate or have withdrawal symptoms usually have developed opioid tolerance, dependence or addiction.[1] The extent of withdrawal will vary significantly; and often will be dependent on the amount or dose, the frequency and consistency of drug use, the type of drug, as well as users' comorbidities such as psychiatric or cognitive disorders, other substance use disorders or dependencies, to mention a few.

Patients or users of opioids who are in withdrawal will have a range of discomfort from very mild to severe. However, most withdrawals are not deemed life-threatening, and even severe cases can be managed appropriately. Although this is generally true, patients or users often have so much anxiety and fear associated with the symptoms that they will do whatever they can to obtain more drugs to relieve the uncomfortable feelings associated with withdrawal.

Withdrawal may be early or late. Early withdrawal may begin about six to 12 hours for short-acting opioids, for example, hydrocodone; or more up to 30 hours after the last dose for longer-acting opioids such as methadone.

These symptoms of withdrawal may last from four to 10 days or up to 21 days and are considered the acute phase of withdrawal.[2,3] However, some patients may still have symptoms that persist long after the acute phase is considered over. These protracted symptoms have been described or called **Post-Acute Withdrawal Syndrome (PAWS) or chronic withdrawal**. These symptoms may continue to last for months with the possibility of associated anxiety, depression, fatigue, etc.

The Early and Late Withdrawal Symptoms

Early withdrawal symptoms

➢ Dilated pupils – vision problems
➢ Muscle aches and pain
➢ Tearfulness
➢ Runny nose
➢ Agitation/Anxiety
➢ Weakness
➢ Sweating
➢ Insomnia.

Late withdrawal symptoms

➢ Nausea and vomiting
➢ Abdominal pain
➢ Diarrhea
➢ Dilated pupils
➢ Tachycardia – increased heart rate
➢ Increased blood pressure
➢ Increase anxiety and irritability
➢ Increased craving
➢ Difficulty urinating
➢ Chills

Giving or Administering Naloxone to
Someone who has Overdosed on Opioids

Naloxone, also called **Narcan**, will save lives if administered quickly and on time. This usually cannot be administered by the victim as he or she would likely be unconscious. This must be administered by a friend, family member, or anyone who has it ready to go when that need arises. Moreover, this need will arise particularly for those on a significant opioid dose and are probably addicted. This is also useful for users of opioids who have significant medical problems (comorbidities), e.g., related to the lungs (pulmonary) or kidneys (renal).

It is expected that people who are overdosing or dying from an overdose are those who are frequent users and are classified as opioid-dependent or drug- dependent and suffering from opioid use disorder or addiction.

However, it is important to understand that anyone can and will die from the use of opioids because of accidental overdose (which is what happens in most overdoses, even for illegal users). Many users who in no way use opioids illegally or outside the normal or recommended way could die. They may sometime have a very low tolerance for opioids, hence the recommendation to start all opioid-naïve patients (when warranted) on low-dose opioids and increase slowly as tolerated. Also, it is rarely ever necessary to start naïve opioid patients on long-acting or extended-release formulations.

It is extremely important that all patients and users of opioids use their medications only as prescribed. Simply put, never assume that two pills are better than one in relieving your pain. That extra pill may be all that is required to put you in opioid-overdose status which may lead to death. The same principle applies to older patients and individuals who are using opioids, particularly those with multiple medical problems requiring the need to take multiple medications.

It is also very important to understand that although it is more likely for those users who have developed opioid tolerance, dependence or addiction to die from an overdose, anyone can and will die.

In other words, an individual does not have to be an addict or opioid use disorder patient to die from an opioid overdose.

Deaths from overdose are not generally dependent on who you are as individuals; rather, it is determined by the amount of opioids that is just enough to shut down users' central nervous system and kill them. Remember that in the end, we are all different, although we may have so much in common.

Avoid taking opioids together with alcohol and/or benzos such as Xanax, Valium, clonazepam, etc. These are deadly combinations.[7,8,9]

Before Administering Naloxone

For everyone taking care of individuals considered potential victims of an opioid overdose, please check the following:

a. Find out if the patient is okay simply by asking "are you okay," giving them a sternal (chest) rub, painful stimuli or shake them.

b. If there is no response, call 911, or have someone else do it if you are not alone.

c. If you have naloxone on hand, administer it to the patient.

d. If the person does not regain consciousness or has no pulse, you may start cardiopulmonary resuscitation (CPR) if you're trained to do that. If there is still no response, you may give the patient another dose of naloxone after every two or three minutes for intramuscular injection, or every three to five minutes for nasal application.

e. Continue CPR until emergency medical services (EMS) arrive.

f. If for whatever reason, EMS has not responded or you are in an area that could not be reached, and the patient recovered but then had a reversal of overdose, you may repeat these injections in one to two hours.

Naloxone comes available in four forms of administration: **subcutaneous**, **intravenous**, **intranasal** and **intramuscular**. Intramuscular and intranasal are the two forms often used in most cases of accidental overdoses, where the drugs are usually administered by a layperson or even healthcare service personnel. Also, the intramuscular and intranasal forms are available in many different packages or kits. This is often determined by the manufacturers, suppliers or pharmaceutical companies responsible for distributing and selling the products.

The two forms of administration are as follows:

1. **Naloxone** in its generic form is sold as **Naloxone Nasal Spray**.

a. Naloxone Nasal Spray is a pre-packaged syringe allowing for nasal route dispensing. This requires minor assembling of the syringe and medication.

The naloxone box usually contains a specialized syringe (specialized Luer- Lock Prefilled Syringe) with pre-filled naloxone tubular glass cartridge (Figure 1). The cartridge containing the naloxone is gentle screwed into the barrel of the syringe, as shown below (**How to Give Nasal Spray Naloxone**). The small cone-shaped device (called **atomizer** – generally sold separately) is gently screwed onto the end of the syringe that will be inserted into each nostril (Figure 2).

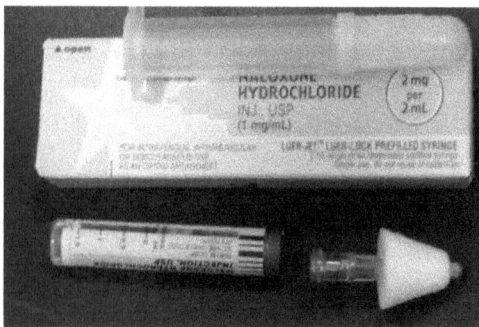
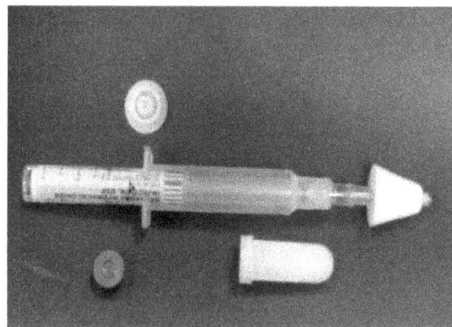

Figure 1   *Figure 2*

How to Give Nasal Spray Naloxone

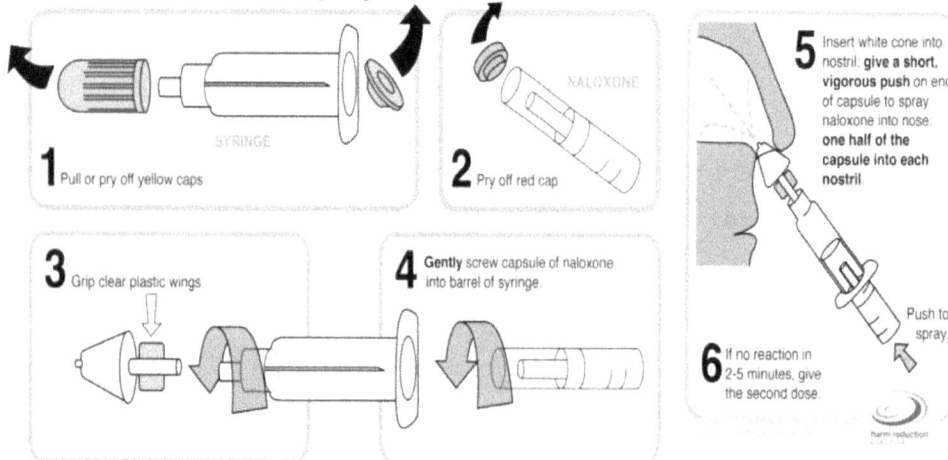

How to give nasal naloxone: Courtesy of Harm Reduction Coalition.[19] Visit them at http://harmreduction.org/.

b. **Naloxone** is packaged and sold as **Narcan Nasal Spray** which is sprayed into the nostril. **No assembling required**.

Instructions for Use
NARCAN (nar′ kan)
(naloxone hydrochloride)

Nasal Spray You and your family members or caregivers should read the Instructions for Use that comes with NARCAN Nasal Spray before using it. Talk to your healthcare provider if you and your family members or caregivers have any questions about the use of NARCAN Nasal Spray.

Use NARCAN Nasal Spray for known or suspected opioid overdose in adults and children.

Important: For use in the nose only.

- **Do not remove or test the NARCAN Nasal Spray until ready to use.**
- **Each NARCAN Nasal Spray has 1 dose and cannot be reused.**
- **You do not need to prime NARCAN Nasal Spray.**

How to use NARCAN Nasal Spray:

Step 1. Lay the person on their back to receive a dose of NARCAN Nasal Spray.

Step 2. Remove NARCAN Nasal Spray from the box. Peel back the tab with the circle to open the NARCAN Nasal Spray.

Step 3. Hold the NARCAN Nasal Spray with your thumb on the bottom of the plunger and your first and middle fingers on either side of the nozzle.

Step 4. Tilt the person's head back and provide support under the neck with your hand. Gently insert the tip of the nozzle into **one nostril** until your fingers on either side of the nozzle are against the bottom of the person's nose.

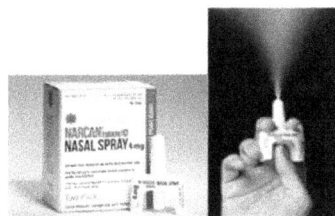

(Photos inserted)

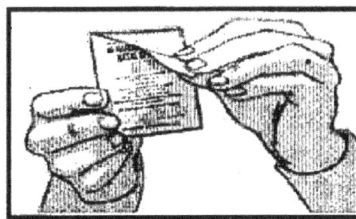

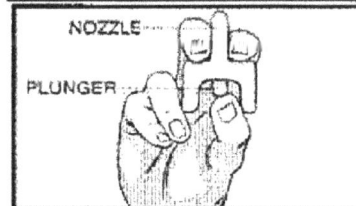

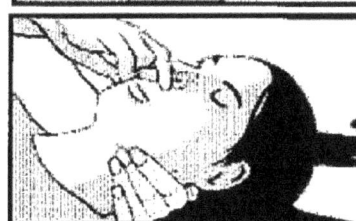

Step 5. Press the plunger firmly to give the dose of NARCAN Nasal Spray.

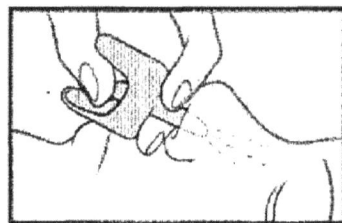

Step 6. Remove the NARCAN Nasal Spray from the nostril after giving the dose.

What to do after NARCAN Nasal Spray has been used:

Step 7. Get emergency medical help right away.

- Move the person on their side (recovery position) after giving NARCAN Nasal Spray.

- Watch the person closely.

- If the person does not respond by waking up, to voice or touch, or breathing normally another dose may be given. NARCAN Nasal Spray may be dosed every 2 to 3 minutes, if available.

- Repeat **Steps 2 through 6** using a new NARCAN Nasal Spray to give another dose in the other nostril. If additional NARCAN Nasal Sprays are available, Steps 2 through 6 may be repeated every 2 to 3 minutes until the person responds or emergency medical help is received.

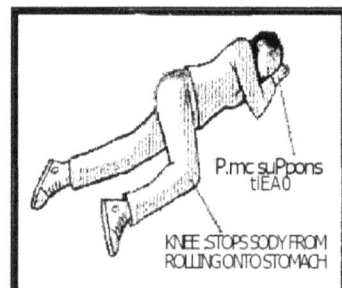

Step 8. Put the used NARCAN Nasal Spray back into its box.

Step 9. Throw away (dispose of) the used NARCAN Nasal Spray in a place that is away from children.

How should I store NARCAN Nasal Spray?

- Store NARCAN Nasal Spray at room temperature between 59°F to 77°F (15°C to 25°C). NARCAN Nasal Spray may be stored for short periods up to 104°F (40°C).
- Do not freeze NARCAN Nasal Spray.
- Keep NARCAN Nasal Spray in the box until ready to use. Protect from light.
- Replace NARCAN Nasal Spray before the expiration date on the box.

Keep NARCAN Nasal Spray and all medicines out of the reach of children.

This Instructions for Use has been approved by the U.S. Food and Drug Administration.

Distributed by Adapt Pharma, Inc. Radnor, PA 19087 USA.

For more information, go to www.narcannasalspray.com or call 1-844-4NARCAN (1-844-462-7226).[4] Issued: 02/2017

❋ NARCAN® (naloxone HCl)
NASAL SPRAY

QUICK START GUIDE
Opioid Overdose Response Instructions

Use NARCAN Nasal Spray (naloxone hydrochloride) for known or suspected opioid overdose in adults and children.
Important: For use in the nose only.
Do not remove or test the NARCAN Nasal Spray until ready to use.

1 Identify Opioid Overdose and Check for Response

Ask person if he or she is okay and shout name.

Shake shoulders and firmly rub the middle of their chest.

Check for signs of opioid overdose:
• Will not wake up or respond to your voice or touch
• Breathing is very slow, irregular, or has stopped
• Center part of their eye is very small, sometimes called "pinpoint pupils"
Lay the person on their back to receive a dose of NARCAN Nasal Spray.

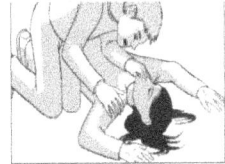

2 Give NARCAN Nasal Spray

Remove NARCAN Nasal Spray from the box.
Peel back the tab with the circle to open the NARCAN Nasal Spray.

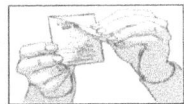

Hold the NARCAN nasal spray with your thumb on the bottom of the plunger and your first and middle fingers on either side of the nozzle.

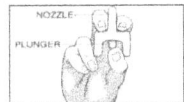

Gently insert the tip of the nozzle into either nostril.
• Tilt the person's head back and provide support under the neck with your hand. Gently insert the tip of the nozzle into **one nostril**, until your fingers on either side of the nozzle are against the bottom of the person's nose.

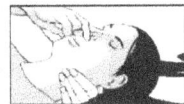

Press the plunger firmly to give the dose of NARCAN Nasal Spray.
• Remove the NARCAN Nasal Spray from the nostril after giving the dose.

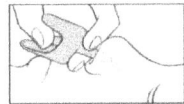

Get emergency medical help right away.

3 Call for emergency medical help, Evaluate, and Support

Move the person on their side (recovery position) after giving NARCAN Nasal Spray.

Watch the person closely.

If the person does not respond by waking up, to voice or touch, or breathing normally another dose may be given. NARCAN Nasal Spray may be dosed every 2 to 3 minutes, if available.

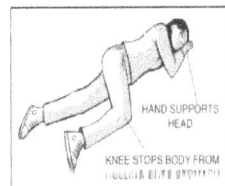

Repeat **Step 2** using a new NARCAN Nasal Spray to give another dose in the other nostril. If additional NARCAN Nasal Sprays are available, repeat step 2 every 2 to 3 minutes until the person responds or emergency medical help is received.

For more information about NARCAN Nasal Spray, go to www.narcannasalspray.com, or call 1-844-4NARCAN (1-844-462-7226).

©2015 ADAPT Pharma, Inc. NARCAN® is a registered trademark licensed to ADAPT Pharma Operations Limited. A1009.01

ADAPT PHARMA

Courtesy of Adapt Pharma Visit https://www.narcan.com/ for more information:[4]

2. The injectable forms of intramuscular naloxone injections:

a. **By attaching the needle to a syringe** requiring users to **load naloxone from a vial (or ampoule)** for injection into the muscle. The needle is usually about one-and-a-half inches long and thick enough to pierce the skin easily (size is about 25 gauge to size 22 gauge); a 3ml syringe is usually adequate. The naloxone is **then injected into any available muscles** (usually thighs or deltoid, in the shoulder). This overall is very simple but requires three steps to set up and administer the medication.

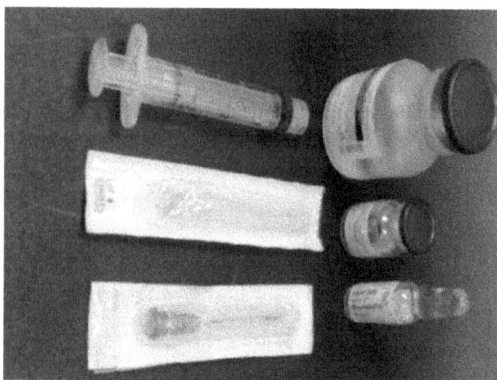

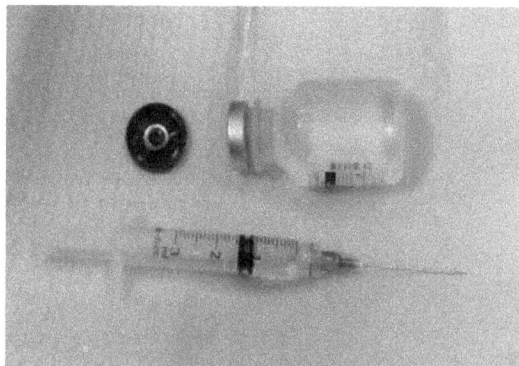

b. **By preloading a filled and ready-to-use syringe**:

There are many variations in this category depending on packaging. The **syringe may come loaded with naloxone ready to attach to the needle and inject,** as in Step A above. This is simple and practical in the case of overdose that a layperson could use. However, other forms of preloaded syringes include naloxone in special cartridges similar to what is used in generic Naloxone Nasal Spray. These prefilled naloxone cartridges usually require an additional device such as Carpuject (a syringe device where naloxone or other medication cartridges are placed in and injected from) to administer the meditation not necessarily by intramuscular route. This is also not generally intended to be used by a layperson, but rather in a hospital or clinic setting to treat opioid overdose.

c. **By autoinjector**, the naloxone is administered by the person giving the auto- injection into a muscle. See below – the product is **Evzio,** accompanied with illustrations of injections. The administrator of the naloxone receives step by step audio instructions from the medication device (**Evzio**) on how to inject the medication in real time.

How to Use EVZIO

Step 1. Pull EVZIO from the outer case. See Figure B.

Figure B

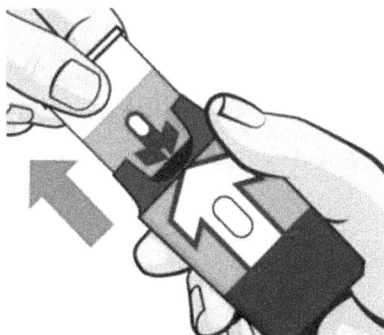

Do not go to Step 2 (Do not remove the **Red** safety guard) until you are ready to use EVZIO. **If you are not ready to use EVZIO, put it back in the outer case for later use.**

Step 2. Pull off the **Red** safety guard. See <u>Figure C</u>.

To reduce the chance of an accidental injection, do not touch the **Black** base of the auto-injector, which is where the needle comes out.

Figure C

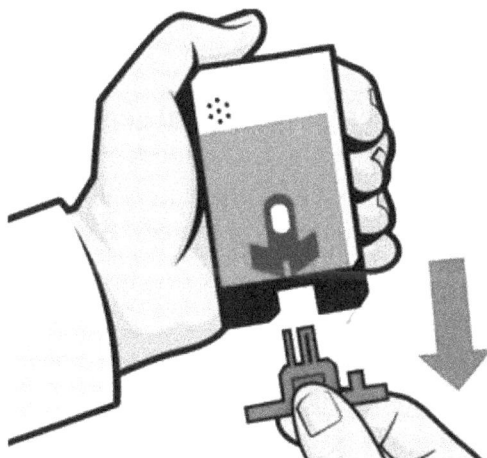

If an accidental injection happens, get medical help right away.

Note: The **Red** safety guard is made to fit tightly. **Pull firmly to remove. Do not replace the Red safety guard after it is removed.**

Step 3. Place the **Black** end of EVZIO against the outer thigh, through clothing, if needed. **Press firmly** and hold in place for 5 seconds. See Figure D.

If you give EVZIO to an infant less than 1 year old, pinch the middle of the outer thigh before you give EVZIO and continue to pinch while you give EVZIO.

Figure D

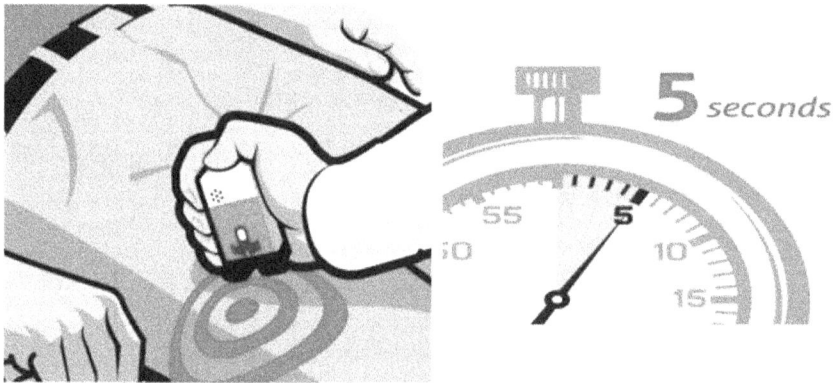

Note: EVZIO makes a distinct sound (click and hiss) when it is pressed against the thigh. This is normal and means that EVZIO is working correctly. Keep EVZIO firmly pressed on the thigh for 5 seconds after you hear the click and hiss sound. The needle will inject and then retract back up into the EVZIO auto-injector and is not visible after use.

Step 4. After using EVZIO, get emergency medical help right away. If symptoms return after an injection with EVZIO, an additional injection using another EVZIO auto-injector may be needed. Give additional injections using a new EVZIO auto- injector every 2 to 3 minutes and continue to closely watch the person until emergency help is received. **EVZIO does not take the place of emergency medical care.**

EVZIO cannot be reused. After use, place the auto-injector back into its outer

case. Do not replace the **Red** safety guard.

Courtesy of Kaléo Pharma. Visit: https://www.evzio.com/patient/ for more information.[18]

Above are some illustrations of injections

The Effect of Naloxone or Narcan

The effect of Naloxone or Narcan is immediate, and will literally bring the comatose or unconscious users back to life if they're not too far gone. Sometimes, additional doses are required to accomplish full consciousness. This may be given if there is no significant response after two to three minutes for intramuscular injections or three to five minutes for nasal applications. Once consciousness is attained, the user should be transferred to an emergency facility and is likely to remain conscious for one-half to one-and-a-half hours for adults, and about three hours for neonates, before the naloxone starts wearing off.

It is important to note that **naloxone will not revive everyone who has a drug overdose; this drug is primarily used for opioid overdoses**. In addition, it may only work poorly or not work at all on opioids that are illegally synthesized, e.g., designer drugs or analog products. In fact, some opioids and known and unknown synthetic analogs have a much longer duration of action on the brain and central nervous system than naloxone (that is, they have a longer half-life than naloxone). But it is still worth having naloxone available for drug overdoses, particularly when you are aware that the user is likely to have taken opioids. It is also still highly recommended to get naloxone regardless of the type of opioid overdose, even though multiple doses may be required to reverse the effects.

A Few Words on the Prescription of Naloxone

Before prescribing naloxone as a provider, it is important to understand the different formulations and packaging associated with naloxone. The purpose of prescribing naloxone to patients is to allow someone in their presence to be able to use it for potential or suspected opioid overdoses. This is not intended for the EMS personnel to use should they visit you. It would be expected that they would bring their own naloxone to the scene.

Naloxone should be ready for use immediately once a potential opioid overdose is detected or suspected. It is also important that whatever form the naloxone is available in, the person who is going to administer it clearly understands how it should be used. Also, make sure that all the components of the package required to administer the naloxone are present.

I've seen naloxone dispensed from pharmacies given to patients to take home in a vial, with no sensible way for those patients or their loved ones to use it in case there is an emergency. In other words, there is no syringe/needle or any feasible way for a layperson to administer the naloxone in case of an emergency. Therefore, if you are a pharmacist dispensing naloxone and the order was written incorrectly, or the naloxone that you have is not ready and capable of being administered by the person or their associates or loved ones, please take that extra step of calling the prescriber to ensure that whatever the patients receive will be useful. It is also important that if your doctor or provider prescribes naloxone for you or your loved ones, make sure that whatever you receive, you understand what it is and how you will be able to use it safely.

Moreover, as prescribers, we have the responsibility to ensure that once we prescribe naloxone to the individual, we must explain what we have prescribed to them and follow-up once they have received it, making sure that they do understand what it is they have received, how it should be administered, and when.

With respect to dispensing naloxone in general, there appears to be a simple fix: ensure that pharmacists dispense only naloxone or naloxone kits ready to be used with all the necessary components rather than dispensing vials of naloxone that are virtually unusable for a layperson.

Naloxone should also be kept safely at appropriate room temperature, without significant sunlight or freezing or cold temperatures. Plus, one should be aware of its expiration date at the time of purchase so that the medication remains current.

Cost of Naloxone

As indicated above, naloxone comes in different formulations and packaging.
- The intramuscular version with vial and syringe price ranges from about $15-$50.
- Narcan Nasal Spray price ranges from about $120 to $150.
- Intramuscular Evzio price ranges from about $4000-$5000.

These are all estimated retail prices. There are also coupons or other discounts that are sometimes offered by pharmaceutical companies. If you have healthcare insurance, in some instances, you will be able to obtain one of these products depending on your coverage; your policy will determine your cost.

You can also check the specific products' websites for further details. Also, other websites are available that will give you general information and, sometimes coupons or discount. Two popular websites are GoodRx.com and Cover my meds.com.[10,20]

Where Does One Go to Get Naloxone?

The fact that naloxone is so crucial and indispensable in the fight against the opioid epidemic by being the drug that saves lives makes its importance impossible to overstate. It has literally saved hundreds of thousands of lives. If this option were not available, the result of the catastrophe that we are now facing would be unimaginable. Many states and federal government agencies have realized the importance of having naloxone available and made more accessible so that the public/consumers can have it any time and lives can be saved.

Naloxone Access Laws

Legislations have been passed in all 50 states and the District of Columbia with the intention of making naloxone more accessible to the public. In some states, no prescription is required from doctor/healthcare providers, and it may be dispensed by pharmacists. Some states require training and/or various stipulations or rules under which naloxone can be administered by members of the general public. Each state has its own version of their access law; there are many similarities as well as variations between the laws. As the opioid epidemic becomes significant, there have been amendments and changes in different state laws to make naloxone more available.[11,12,13,14,15]

The Good Samaritan Laws

Most states and the District of Columbia have passed Good Samaritan laws, which are generally designed to protect individuals from arrest or prosecution if they report a drug overdose or administer life-saving measures to someone who may have overdosed illegally or legally. In some instances, both the overdose victim and the person(s) administering life-saving measures may be eligible for or granted immunity from arrest and prosecution for the use or possession of illegal drugs/opioids. The Good Samaritan laws are designed to save lives as opposed to criminalizing those involved in what are probably criminal activities involving opioid use.

The opioid epidemic has been gaining more support for a treatment- oriented approach rather than law enforcement application or criminalizing the people involved.[16,17]

On March 16, 2018, the Trump administration indicated that they are considering several options including the death penalty for major drug dealers. How such legislation will impact the Good Samaritan laws, and others is left to be seen.

For both the Good Samaritan laws as well as the Naloxone Access laws, it is highly recommended that you check and be informed of your state's laws and regulations and what is required of you.[17]

Naloxone can, therefore, be obtained from your local pharmacies; check within your states to see what is required. If no prescription is required, you may purchase it over-the-counter at your local pharmacy. There are also available **MAT programs** that may provide naloxone or can advise you where to go. I've also included a list of useful government agencies, associations and websites that can further help concerning acquiring naloxone, as well as other useful resources that may be helpful when you need them (**Useful Resources and Websites**).

Naloxone is also crucial if you are taking care of an older adult or anyone with other medical problems with significant opioid use. That person does not have to have a drug dependency or be addicted to opioids. Please ensure that you also have naloxone available just in case there's an accidental overdose.

References, Recommended Readings and Resources

1. Drug Enforcement Administration. Drug Facts Sheet-Narcotics. https://www.dea.gov/druginfo/drug_data_sheets/Narcotics.pdf. Accessed July 4, 2018.

2. US National Library of Medline. Opiate and Opioid Withdrawal. Last reviewed April 20, 2016. https://medlineplus.gov/ency/article/000949. htm. Accessed July 2, 2018.

3. Substance Abuse and Mental Health Services Administration. Based on TIP 54. Quick Guide for Clinician. Managing Indictment Chronic Pain in Adults with or in Recovery from Substance Use Disorders. Published 2012. https://store.samhsa.gov/shin/content/SMA13-4792/SMA13-4792.pdf. Accessed July 2, 2018.

4. Narcan: Visit: wvvw.narcannasalspray.com for more information.

5. Naloxone: Visit: www.naloxon.com for more information.

6. Evzio: Visit: wvvw.evzio.com for more information.

7. Benzodiazepines and Opioids | National Institute on Drug Abuse (NIDA). March 2018. https://www.drugabuse.gov/drugs-abuse/ opioids/benzodiazepines-opioids. Accessed June 10, 2018.

8. Centers for Disease Control and Prevention (CDC). National Vital Statistics System, Mortality. CDC WONDER Online Database. https://wonder.cdc. gov/. Published 2017.

9. NIH. National Institute of Drug Abuse. Overdose Death Rates. https://www.drugabuse.gov/related-topics/trends-statistics/overdose-death- rates. Accessed June 4, 2018.

10. How GoodRx Works. Learn how to save up to 80% on your prescriptions. https://www.goodrx.com/naloxone?drug- name=naloxone. Accessed July 22, 2018.

11. CDC Newsroom. Expanding Naloxone use could reduce drug overdose deaths and save lives. April 24, 2015. https://www.cdc.gov/media/releas- es/2015/p0424-naloxone.html. Accessed April 16, 2018.

12. Preventing the Consequences of Opioid Overdose: Understanding Naloxone Access Laws. https://www.samhsa.gov/capt/sites/default/files/resources/naloxone-access-laws-tool.pdf. Accessed March 16, 2018.

13. Susan P Weinstein Commentary: Naloxone Access and Good Samaritan Overdose Protection Laws Abound in State Legislatures. June 24, 2015. https://drugfree.org/learn/drug-and-alcohol-news/ commentary-naloxone- access-good-samaritan-overdose-protection- laws-abound-state-legislatures/. Accessed March 16, 2018.

14. Jerome M. Adams, MD, MPH, VADM. Increasing Naloxone Awareness and Use: The Role of Health Care Practitioners. 15. JAMA. 2018;319(20):2073-2074. May 22/29, 2018. https://jamanetwork.com/journals/jama/article-abstract/2678206. Accessed on June 30, 2018.

15. Francie Diep. How easy is it to get naloxone in your states? Here's how states have made it easier for bystanders to administer naloxone to overdose victims. April 6, 2018. https://psmag.com/news/how-easy- is-it-to-get-naloxone-in-your-state. Accessed on June 30,2018.

16. The Network for Public Health Law. Legal Interventions to Reduce Over- dose Mortality: Naloxone Access and Overdose Good Samaritan Law. https://www.networkforphl.org/_asset/qz5pvn/legal-interventions-to-re- duce-overdose.pdf. Accessed March 16,2018.

17. Menu of State Laws Related to Prescription Drug Overdose Emergencies. https://www.cdc.gov/phlp/docs/menu-pdoe.pdf. Accessed March 30, 2018.

18. Kaléo Pharma. Visit: https://www.evzio.com/patient/ for more information.

19. Harm Reduction Coalition. http://harmreduction.org/. Last visited August 17, 2018.

20. Cover My Meds https://www.covermymeds.com/main/about/ Last visited July 22, 2018.

Chapter 12
The Challenges of Managing Chronic Pain Patients with Opioids who have Psychiatric and/or-Non-Opioid Substance Use Disorders

Mental Illness or Psychiatric Disorder Patients Need Opioids Too

Mental illness or psychiatric disorders are often considered among the most undertreated, unrecognized or undiagnosed medical conditions. In addition, when diagnoses are made, very often adequate treatment is not provided. These problems are compounded by the shortage of mental health providers such as psychiatrists as well as other clinical providers.

It was reported that 51% of all opioid prescriptions are written for to adults with mental health conditions or disorders, which make up about 16% of those with mental illness.[2,7]

In 2014, a National Survey on Drug Use and Health had revealed that 43.6 million people (18.1% of the US population) experienced some form of mental illness disorder. In addition, 20.2 million people (8.4%) had a substance use disorder; and 7.9 million had both, referred to as co-occurring mental illness and substance use disorder.[8] These statistics are significant in light of the fact that individuals with mental disorders are generally among the most difficult to treat for pain

Individuals who Use or Abuse Illegal Substances

Individuals who use or abuse illegal substances such as cocaine, methamphetamine, PCP, marijuana, etc.; or other diverted legal medications, for example, Xanax and Soma also complicate the issue with respect to opioids use and abuse. In addition, alcohol use and abuse also add to the challenges faced in the opioid epidemic.[3]

The presence of mental illnesses and/or substance abuse provides a common challenge in pain management. As pain management specialists, we must balance the risks of giving or not giving opioids to patients who have significant mental disorders, even if they are currently on medication and under the care of their psychiatrists/counselors. Patients with mental health disorders are more likely to abuse opioids; it is not surprising that there is a higher demand for opioids from those who have mental illness compared to the general population. This demand for opioids is more significant in patients with mental illness than those without. They correspondingly received the highest percentage of opioids prescribed in the country. They are, of course, just like anyone else, patients with mental illness who have pain and must be treated appropriately. This requires, in the case of those with significant mental health problems, the need to have complete coordination of medical care between psychiatric and psychological service providers and pain management specialists.

These patients need to be monitored very closely, particularly when they are taking medications that may compound the adverse effects of opioids. These medications include (but are not limited to) benzos. Use of other substances such as alcohol should be off-limits. Patients and their caregivers or loved ones need to be educated with a greater emphasis on the use of opioids and possible drug interactions/substances that could have serious adverse effects.

Pain Management Practices May Not Prescribe Opioids to Anyone who is Currently Using Illicit Drugs

As a general rule, most pain management practices may not prescribe opioids to anyone who is currently using illicit drugs such as cocaine, marijuana, methamphetamine, etc. Patients are typically discharged if they are found to be using any of these illegal drugs while on opioids. This applies to all patients; the risks are even higher for patients with mental disorders.

Marijuana sometimes may be treated differently by some practices depending on which part of the country they are located. However, it is worthwhile to remember for those of us who have DEA licenses that our prescription license is given by the federal government, and not the state in which we practice. Currently, marijuana still remains illegal according to federal government laws.

Patients who are on opioids for a prolonged period and become opioid dependents or addicts will probably develop depression and/or associated anxiety. Some of them may have developed these disorders related to the need or compulsion to obtain drugs. If they do have a mental illness, then at times they take the opioids in an attempt to alleviate symptoms related to their mental disorders, rather than for pain.

This population also requires more care and a management approach requiring the interdisciplinary facilitation of their care. Pain patients who are addicts or substance-dependent, whether it be opioids or psychiatric medications or unknown illegal drugs, remain one of the more difficult groups of patients to be treated. They will require both aggressive therapy for addictions as well as for mental health, along with all the supporting opinions/services required to facilitate their treatment.

Patients Can and Indeed Do Well with Mental Disorders

An important point to be made is that there is a significant number of patients diagnosed with mental disorders, most commonly depression and anxiety. The vast majority of these patients can and indeed do well when managed and monitored appropriately in most pain management settings.

There are always even greater challenges for patients who have multiple psychiatric disorders in addition to depression and/or anxiety, such as bipolar disorder and/or schizophrenia. In addition, it is also challenging if they have poor social structures, limited financial resources, inadequate education, etc. It is often best to take each patient one at a time, determine his or her needs, and find the best way to administer treatment.

Unfortunately, not every patient is suitable for pain management and or opioid prescriptions. Sometimes, as physicians/healthcare providers, our best option is to say we cannot help you.

If the patient's circumstances allow us to help, we can direct them on a path that would be more meaningful for their overall treatment and/or recovery.

Opioid Overdose – How Many Are Real Suicides?

The question often arises regarding how many deaths attributed to unintentional opioid overdoses are truly unintentional, as opposed to suicide-by-opioid. The debates have continued as it is virtually impossible to determine whether some of these victims are actually the results of suicides.

The CDC has noted a rise in suicide rate: by 24% between 1999 and 2014, from 10.5 deaths per 100,000 people to 13 per 100,000. However, a significant number of these drug-related fatal overdoses were reported or classified as undetermined.[4,5]

References, Recommended Readings and Resources

1. Bruce Japsen. Psychiatrist Shortage Escalates as U.S. Mental Health Needs Grow. February 25, 2018. https://www.forbes.com/sites/ bruce-japsen/2018/02/25/psychiatrist-shortage-escalates-as-u-s-mental-health- needs-grow/#28e059ff1255. Accessed 05/17/2018.

2. Matthew A. Davis, MPH, Ph.D., Lewei A. Lin, MD, Haiyin Liu, MA, and Brian D. Sites, MD, MS. Prescription Opioid Use among Adults with Mental Health Disorders in the United States. June 26, 2017, https://kaiserhealthnews.files.wordpress.com/2017/06/opioidembargo- article.pdf. Accessed August 2, 2018.

3. Puja Seth, Ph.D.; Lawrence Scholl, Ph.D.; Rose A. Rudd, MSPH; Sarah Bacon, Ph.D., *MMMWR.* Overdose deaths involving opioids, cocaine, and psychostimulants – United States, 2015-2016. https://www.cdc.gov/ mmwr/volumes/67/wr/mm6712a1.htm. Accessed May 5, 2018.

4. Maria A. Oquendo, M.D., Ph.D., and Nora D. Volkow, Suicide: Silent Contributor to Opioid Overdose Deaths. N Engl J Med 2018; 378:1567-1569. April 26, 2018. https://www.nejm.org/doi/ full/10.1056/NEJMp1801417. Accessed May 26, 2018.

5. Stone DM, Holland KM, Bartholow B, E Logan J, LiKamWa McIntosh W, TrudeauA, Rockett IRH. Deciphering suicide and other manners of death associated with drug intoxication: A Center for Disease Control and Prevention consultation meeting summary. Am J Public Health 2017;107:1233- 1239. https://www.ncbi.nlm.nih.gov/ pubmed/28640689. Accessed May 26, 2018.

6. Brigitte Manteuffel Shannon CrossBear. Caregiver Guide Substance Use Disorder Treatment Planning for Youth with Co-Occurring Disorders. https:// www.air.org/sites/default/files/downloads/report/ Substance_Abuse_Care- giver_Guide_Jan%202015.pdf. Last visited August 21, 2018.

7. Brian Sites, MD. Why Are Patients with Mental Health Disorders Getting More Opioids? Jul 14, 2017. https://www.asra.com/news/164/ why-are-pa- tients-with-mental-health-diso. Accessed August 22, 2018.

8. Rachel N. Lipari, Ph.D., and Struther L. VanHorn, M.A. Trends in Substance Use Disorders among Adults Aged 18 and Older. June 29, 2017. https:// www.samhsa.gov/data/sites/default/files/report_2790/ShortReport-2790.html. Accessed August 22, 2018.

Part Three
SOLUTIONS, PREVENTION
AND TRYING TO FIND OUR WAY OUT OF
THE OPIOID EPIDEMIC

Chapter 13

You Dare Not Test My Child for Drugs!

I've heard it said once or several times that one of the most significant mental or psychological traumas that parents can go through is the loss of a child. The expectation is that you will transition and your child will put you to rest. However, what happens when a child unexpectedly passed because of the opioid epidemic? Moreover, how can you reduce the risks of that happening?

The option of testing children in schools is something worth considering. Notice I said "option." We're still a free society, and we love to have all our independence, our Second Amendment rights, civil rights, all the rights given to us by the Constitution and, of course, our Almighty God. Exercising your right to raise your child the way you want to should ultimately be your responsibility. I hope that I am abundantly clear on that point. I also want to be clear on the fact that all parents/guardians and those responsible for children, adolescents or anyone in their custody must and should realize that regardless of your best intentions and goodwill, sometimes there is a greater force acting against all of that. I've often heard family members and guardians who commented that no one could love their children or the people they are responsible for more than he or she does. There is no reason to doubt the love that they have or that you have for the ones you take care of.

However, it is important that you realize that sometimes, your love and all that you have done don't matter anymore when the ones you care about become addicts. They are no longer the exact representation of who they were before they changed. I know that sometimes it is hard and painful for you to appreciate that because you are in the giving-and-caring mode and you hope that will be understood and reciprocated in actions that reflect an appreciation for your efforts.

The simple truth is those who are addicted or have become addicts have lost or are losing their ability to reciprocate the goodness you have given and, as such, are in no position to be the person you thought they were. In other words, sometimes love just isn't enough.[1,2,3]

Random and optional drug testing for your child may provide you an option for early intervention should your child test positive for opioids or illicit drugs. Prevention and early intervention are still among the best options that will significantly reduce the risks of your child or children and our loved ones becoming victims of the opioid epidemic.

It is worthwhile that you also remember that your child doesn't have to be a bad person to become an addict, neither does he or she have to belong to one of "those other people or groups," whomever you perceived them to be. In addition, they aren't planning in the initial stage of drug use to be deceptive or to do things that would be considered unbecoming of him or her with respect to the relationship you share.

Here's another important issue that often comes up: how much or how well do I really know my child? As you struggle like so many who have lost their children, loved ones and others, there is always a common theme that emerges: "if only I knew," if only I realized that they were doing those things, the outcome would have been different. Moreover, yes, you're right!

So how does one get to know those things? First, know your child, children, loved ones and/or significant others well. You should be acutely aware of and so in sync with them to appreciate the changes that emerge. As parents or guardians, your kids or children should have no secrets from you. ***Unfortunately, sometimes we compromise good parenting for so-called independence and free will***. There are parents who have never been in their children's rooms or "areas that the children use almost exclusively," not just for weeks, but probably for years. Moreover, when they do go in, they only do a quick glance, then they're on their way.

I encourage parents and guardians to be a part of your children's lives and their world. Don't wait until they are 15, 16 or 17 years old before you start getting curious about what they're doing in their room or in "their space." Simply put, be nosy with your children, for you are responsible for their well- being. They may not know it now, but they will understand it later.

Your children will undoubtedly change right in front of your eyes as they grow and evolve into puberty, into their teenage years and into early adulthood. There's often nothing unusual going on but be aware of changes that imply or suggest regression from what your children are accustomed to doing or being. For example: what if your daughter was one of the best-dressed people around, and suddenly her hair or nails or even general hygiene and grooming are not that important anymore or are gradually fading in importance?

Try to find answers as to why that might be; these could be symptoms of a more significant problem such as drug use, the onset of psychiatric illness, physical and or sexual abuse. Similarly, your son may follow a similar path, or your children's friends and associates may also be changing and becoming different from who they were to completely new and different persons.

The friends and company your kids keep is another important factor. It is imperative for you to have a good sense of who they are, where they live, and who lives in their vicinity so that when your child visits (if you permit) them, you will feel comfortable knowing that they are likely to be safe. You may know, for example, that John or Mary's mother is a wonderful person, which is great! However, how about the spouse and their siblings? What about their neighbors who usually visit? Do you know them, do you trust them, or do you even care?

Don't be afraid to do the math. If your child or their friends have cars, things or gifts that their income does not support, it is mandatory that you know and understand why that's possible. Very simply, your child's friend may not be a drug user, but he may be selling it, which is even worse. So, your child or your children may be just a short way from "just try this."

It is so easy to think that if you're a good person who has done everything almost right or entirely right, and your kids and family are the same, it is only reasonable to expect that only good things will happen to you and your family. However, the opioid epidemic does not respect good and bad families; it does not discriminate by race or class or sex or religion.

Once you're caught up, or get hooked having a good time, you are on track for opioid addiction and all the destruction and possible deaths that come with it.

Indeed, love your children and significant others, but never let that blind you to the reality of an epidemic that is often stronger and more powerful than the love between you and your loved ones.

When Your Little Ones are
All Grown up – and are Now Called Adults

Wow! Certainly, the time has gone by so quickly, and now the little babies have grown to be adults in their late teens or early 20s. They are now in control of their lives and the future that lies ahead.

The opioid epidemic does not make a distinction between adults of any category or teens or adults. Once you become a victim of the opioid epidemic, your lives are dictated by the forces of addiction.

For all the young adults who have escaped path of substance abuse of any kind, you can consider yourself fortunate. In addition, you are also in the majority. You can now take some time to help so many who may not as lucky as you have been.

For those who may not have made it on to college and are working straight out of high school, the temptation for drug use and abuse will always be there. Unfortunately, so many have become victims of opioid use and abuse. The freedom to be in control of one own's life is truly awesome but comes with unlimited responsibilities which, if not properly used, can lead to catastrophic consequences. Sometimes the "potential for easy money" seems great and attractive. But they also often lead to destructive behaviors and addictions for those involved in drugs or illegal substances as a way out of jobs that they do not consider lucrative enough to sustain their desired lifestyle.

For students in college, the challenges are also there. So many students are stressed, fatigued, lacking sleep, are low-energy, and pressured to do well. There is always someone around, sometimes another student, who can fix the problems by providing drugs that are "appropriate," as they see it. This can and often leads to the potential for substance abuse, including but not limited to opioids. It is important that students in college at whatever level be aware of the potential of falling into the trap of "getting help," only to realize that they have been gradually pulled into the path of substance abuse.

If this is not corrected or addressed appropriately, the chance of addiction or substance use disorder is significantly high. Therefore, well- informed and educated students have a better chance of recognizing and avoiding the potential for abuse, and therefore escaping the pitfalls that await the next victims.

"The Good Drugs"

Of course, one doesn't have to be an adult before the challenges of drugs, often described as "things to help us cope" or "the good drugs" come into play. Unfortunately, some kids in their preteens and carly teens are exposed to drugs of some sort, or even smoking cigarettes.

It is very critical in this early stage of our kids' lives to be fully aware of everything that they are doing and are possibly exposed to. Also, awareness of their mental states and actions is critical in assessing changes or variations from what is considered their normal status. It is so important to continually remind them not to take any substances, candies, sweets, drinks or pills or whatever form the so- called good drugs or substances are presented to them. Our kids at all times should know everything and be responsible for everything that they consume or ingest.

This doesn't have to be opioids, cocaine, marijuana or any of the significant known illegal drugs. It is still vital that they know and feel entirely comfortable and be responsible for everything that they ingest. This sounds very simple at some level, but it is actually critical, particularly when kids go to parties or other people's homes and are unaware of what they are consuming, and simply trust their friends and associates.

It is so important to realize that blind trust is also potentially giving your mind and body to whoever is giving you whatever that might make you feel good.

This can be very dangerous on so many levels, leading to physical, mental, and sexual abuse; or even death. Constantly remind your children and loved ones never to allow themselves to get caught up in the usual free-sampling business, where a sample is given, and once the recipients like it, then it is time to pay. This, of course, is a standard practice used by many pharmaceutical companies for years, or even at friendly stores such as Sam's Club or Costco, where you get to sample a product while browsing through the store before you purchase it. It is on us to teach our children and young adults to take control of their lives and full responsibility for everything they consume at all times.

How Do You Help Your Adult Children?

Being an adult gives one control of one's life and the way one wants to live. This question often comes up: who pays for the life they choose to live? Of course, if they are paying for the lifestyle they choose, it may be considered a very serious interruption if one tries to interject. As parents, it is not uncommon that we will try to do that, even if we fail in the process. Moreover, although our kids may not seem to understand or believe that we know enough or have life experience, common sense eventually prevails in most cases, making the process easier for both parents and students.

However, what if you are the parents financing your adult children in college? Do you have the right to be involved in their lives and help them live a life that is consistent with what you believe to be the norm or appropriate? That's a question you will have to answer. However, bear in mind that your adult children also have the right to determine how they live their lives. For example, if your adult children should become involved in the use of illegal drugs or substances, you do not have the right to know unless they give that information to you. Should they be in counseling for drug use, opioid use or other behavioral or psychiatric issues, you may never know. At the same time, they depend on you to be responsible for their support.

Some parents have taken the position that unless there is full disclosure, then and only then, can support be expected. Others have taken the position that they will support them regardless, or are somewhere in between. Whatever your opinion, please be aware that for you to have access to information about your adult children, they must grant it to you. Being an emergency contact is not the same as them allowing you access to their information. If you are involved in your children's lives, you can help to facilitate and possibly ensure a more meaningful recovery/resolution of the process.

Divorced Parents

The rate of divorce in this country is about 50%. It is certain that there will be children of all ages as well as adults who are children of divorced parents. As stated so many times in this book, the opioid epidemic does not respect anyone's social status, class, or whatever criteria they may apply to consider themselves special.

Children of divorced parents are sometimes the victims of disputes and unreconciled differences between ex-spouses. In some instances, the children may be used as pawns in a fight or a feud they probably have absolutely nothing to do with. Depending on the age of the children, they sometimes can be more prone to be exposed to illegal drugs or substances of abuse; and this can sometimes spiral out of control, resulting in children becoming potential victims of opioids or other addictions.

It is truly of paramount importance, particularly when kids are preadolescents and even adults, that divorced parents really make a concerted effort to put the children's interests above their own personal interests or vendettas. For children who are old enough or mature enough, they sometimes can form a good bridge or a buffer between divorced parents. But usually, those children are probably the ones least likely to be involved in drugs and illegal substances. The ones who are often and most severely affected are the ones with behavioral issues, delayed maturity, or probably added psychological issues directly related to divorce or other factors.

These kids need to be monitored more closely, and again, it is of extreme importance that parents put their kids first instead of their own personal feelings. It is always a bad idea for either parent to try to influence their children to take sides because that often leads to unfortunate decisions and outcomes (although not always).

Some Important Legal Issues Related to Children and
Parents' Rights from Your Medical Doctor – *Therefore, Get Your Own Attorney*

This section of this book addresses many issues related to individual rights and liberty. It is important to realize that each state has its own laws, although some could be similar and/or applied differently per state. In addition, there are also federal laws which govern the application of each action as it applies. I recommend that you refer to the laws of your states, and consult an attorney to ensure that whatever action you take or plan to take is appropriate and legal. Remember that this doesn't have to make sense to you.

I included this section because very often when individuals are involved in drugs and/or have a behavioral issue that is related to drugs or psychiatric illness, they will have the need for appropriate family member support.

It is usually better to establish personnel who will be involved in making healthcare decisions before a healthcare emergency occurs. If no prior decision is made, the responsibility of decision-making will default to the adult child who is ill, who may not at that time have the capacity to fully understand or care for him or herself appropriately.

Generally, to be involved in your children lives at various levels from when they are minors to young adults with respect to their healthcare, well-being and educational performance, there are certain laws and or rules which you will need to become more familiar with. Understanding these laws and how they apply to your particular needs in your state may help you navigate some of the pitfalls that potentially await you should you feel the need to be more involved in your children's lives. Without proper knowledge or understanding, you may be left on the outside looking in, helplessly trying to find solutions. Here are a few things that are important to know.

"**The Family Educational Rights and Privacy Act (FERPA)** (20 U.S.C. § 1232g; 34 CFR Part 99) is a Federal law that protects the privacy of student education records. The law applies to all schools that receive funds under an applicable program of the U.S. Department of Education.

FERPA gives parents certain rights concerning their children's education records. These rights transfer to the student when he or she reaches the age of 18 or attends a school beyond the high school level. Students to whom the rights have transferred are "eligible students."

Therefore, the Privacy Rule generally allows a parent to have access to the medical records about his or her child, as his or her minor child's personal representative when such access is not inconsistent with State or other law.

There are also exceptions to the law." [4,7] Note that the law does not apply to institutions that do not receive funding from the government for applicable educational programs which other schools receive that are subjected to the law. The most important point here is to realize that once your children reach the age of 18, under federal law or wherever applicable, their records and the decisions that they make with those records are theirs.

"The Health Insurance Portability and Accountability Act (HIPAA) is a rule which gives you as well as your now emancipated or young adult children, with few exceptions, the right to inspect, review, and receive a copy of your medical records and billing records that are held by health plans and health care providers covered by the Privacy Rule.

Only the persons, individuals (patients) or their personal representatives have the right to access their records. This right is only given or belong to the person who owns the medical records. You, however, do not have the right to access a provider's psychotherapy notes.

Psychotherapy notes are notes that a mental health professional takes during a conversation with a patient. They are kept separate from the patient's medical and billing records.

HIPAA also does not allow the provider to make most disclosures about psychotherapy notes about you without your authorization.

A health care provider or health plan may send copies of your records to another provider or health plan only as needed for treatment or payment or with your permission. The Privacy Rule does not require the health care provider or health plan to share information with other providers or plans.[4,7]

A provider cannot deny you a copy of your records because you have not paid for the services you have received. However, a provider may charge for the reasonable costs for copying and mailing the records. The provider cannot charge you a fee for searching for or retrieving your records." [4]

With respect to **HIPAA**, it is important to understand that your adult children are now in full control of their medical records. Psychotherapists' or behavioral therapists' medical notes or records can be very important concerning behavioral issues and possible opioid or substance use issues. The challenge and approach that each parent faces will ultimately depend on how you and your children navigate, negotiate or compromise on these issues which they are essentially in control of. Now, you may be in control of other things that are important to them, but they are in control of their medical records. When all is said and done, they are your children, and as a family, you will have to decide how best to deal with these issues. But also remember that if your children are being treated by their favorite school psychotherapist or medical doctor or whoever, and these decisions have not been made before the start of treatment, it is highly unlikely that you will find any professional or institution that will speak to you regarding your children's well- being; unless that was previously established, and you're not just the emergency contact, but someone whose children have entrusted you with their healthcare information.

Of course, if your children decide that they do not wish for you to have access to their information, then that is their right, and their expectation, as well as the law's, is that their wishes will be honored by their healthcare providers.

A **healthcare proxy** (sometimes called a **durable medical power of attorney for healthcare**) is a legal document which stipulates that an agent/ representative or person will make medical decisions in the event that you are unable to do so. This may have limited applicability with respect to what your wishes are, or there may be very specific details outlined in the document.

The designated healthcare agent/ representative may also be entrusted to decide as the need arises during the care of the person they are representing.

A **living will** is a document which outlines what medical treatments you wish to have done should you become incapacitated and unable to decide for yourself. These decisions are usually enforced or supervised by your healthcare proxy or agents. The living will often take the form of your individual preferences, religious beliefs, or cultural inclinations or whatever you deemed appropriate for someone to manage your health when you are unable to do so. For example, you may choose not to be resuscitated (through a Do Not Resuscitate or DNR order) or to be intubated, and you may wish not to receive any blood transfusion regardless of the consequences.

Advance directives are legal documents which may constitute healthcare proxy, living will and/or other documented wishes/orders. Different states have different laws, versions, names, and applications for these directives, although there may also be similarities. The general concepts are the same, but different names may apply to the same thing in different states. Be sure to check your state's laws and/ or attorney to ensure that you have the correct forms/documents and interpretation of its laws as they apply in your particular circumstances and state.[5]

There are two other frequent terms that are often used in dealing with healthcare-related issues regarding privacy and access, as well as treatments. These two terms are **capacity** and **competence.** Capacity refers to one's functional ability to access, analyze, interpret and put into action rational plans as dictated by his or her current condition and/or the factors affecting it. Therefore, one is considered to have capacity if that person is generally believed to have a sound mind, and hence has the capability to direct their well-being. Everyone is given that right of self-determination by the Constitution and is deemed to have the capacity to direct his or her own lives. In all states, everyone, until proven otherwise, has the capacity to direct their own affairs, including medical treatments and personal business. A medical professional/psychiatrist may determine whether an individual has the capacity to function. This is without the need of the court or a court hearing. Of course, the individual who is now deemed incapacitated may contest this legally.

The term **competence** is a legal term and is generally determined by a court of law. If a person lacks the capacity to function normally, that person may be deemed incompetent. However, this will require both legal and medical determination, with the court assessing the situation/evidence and then determining whether an individual is competent are not. This may be related to healthcare matters or other legal issues.

Understanding and at least being somewhat familiar with these terms and laws will help you be more in tune with your loved ones. The last thing you want to happen (as in so many cases) is to be shut out of your children's or your loved ones' lives and be on the outside looking in. These systems and laws, although serving useful purposes, can sometimes take away your children and loved ones from you, so you become the enemy on the outside looking in, unable to do anything meaningful. This is even more critical in young adults who go off to college and sometimes get in the wrong crowd, or just appears to have innocently done the wrong thing.

Now their parents find out there is nothing that they can do as they are denied access to their "kids." This system can literally lock your children away from you.[6]

The need to protect your family, your loved ones and yourself with advanced directives is extremely important. And again, remember that being listed as an emergency contact does not dictate or give clarity to how all your medical or your family's medical issues should be dealt with. This includes privacy issues with respect to **FERPA** and **HIPPA**, and what decisions you and your family are comfortable with.

The importance of access and clarity to you and your family members' medical records can become incredibly important if your family members are willing to let you be a part of their care.

Often in this way, you and your family will know the truth of what is totally and completely involved in your loved one's lives, and be able to take a more rational and meaningful step to recovery. Unfortunately, individuals who are using illegal drugs or substances or are under the influence of medications/drugs often lose the ability to be rational and may become a cognitively different version of the person you knew before.

Although it is best to establish initial expectations going forward regarding individual privacy and who has access to personal records, there is no guarantee that the person you're trying to protect will not change their mind. Moreover, if they do so, they will have the final say in what happens to their medical records, even at their peril and your willingness to help them. In short, your adult children may simply say "I do not want my parents to have any access or any more access whatsoever to my medical records," and that's how it will be legally.

Improve your Contacts and Connections

In the era of the opioid epidemic, every little bit helps with respect to being able to communicate with your loved ones or to have access to them when you need to. Sometimes, when your young adult children leave and go to college or off to a new job, they may be so overwhelmed that communications between you and them may become limited or even non-existent, although this is not typical in most cases. Every parent or guardian needs to establish reliable connections and contact with your children, wherever they may be. This may include but are not limited to, names, phone numbers, email addresses, and even the social media accounts of their friends and associates, as well as their parents' or guardians' information.

If there is the lease of an apartment involved, you should have the information of the landlord and, if possible, anyone who shares an apartment with your children.

Always try to extend the link of contacts involving your children to as many associates as possible. Sometimes, contacts like these can be priceless and may lead to invaluable anonymous information, which may be of significant benefit to you in helping to intervene if necessary, should your children's circumstances dictate that. Of course, each child is different, and each approach to everyone should accordingly be different. However, do whatever it takes to be involved not just with your child or children, but their friends, associates and their families, too.

You will then have multiple points of contact with your loved ones from many different sources, should that ever become necessary.

References, Recommended Readings and Resources

1. National Institute on Drug Abuse. Principles of Drug Addiction Treatment: A Research-Based Guide. Third edition. Last reviewed December 2012. https://www.drugabuse.gov/sites/default/files/ podat_1.pdf. Accessed July 2, 2018.

2. Thomas Kosten, Tony P George. The Neurobiology of Opioid Dependence: Implications for Treatment. NIH. Science & Practice Perspectives. 13-20. August 2002. https://www.researchgate.net/ publication/5288549_The_ eurobiology_of_Opioid_Dependence_ Implications_for_Treatment. Accessed July 7, 2018.

3. Gary Peltz, MD, Ph.D.; Thomas C. Südhof, MD. The Neurobiology of Opioid Addiction and the Potential for Prevention Strategies. *JAMA*. 2018;319(20):2071-2072. May 22/29, 2018. https://jamanetwork.com/ journals/jama/article-abstract/2680118. Accessed June 30, 2018.

4. Health Information Privacy. U.S. Department of Health & Human Ser- vices. https://www.hhs.gov/hipaa/for-professionals/faq/mental- health/in- dex.html. Accessed May 5, 2018.

5. Health Care Proxy Appointing Your Health Care Agent in New York State. https://www.health.ny.gov/publications/1430.pdf. Accessed May 6, 2018.

6. Raphael J. Leo, M.D., Competency and the Capacity to Make Treatment Decisions: A Primer for Primary Care Physicians. https://www.ncbi.nlm. nih.gov/pmc/articles/PMC181079/. Accessed May 10, 2018.

7. Health Information Privacy https://www.hhs.gov/hipaa/for- profession-als/faq/227/can-i-access-medical-record-if-i-have-power-of-attorney/ index.html Accessed October 23, 2018.

Chapter 14

Some Useful and Helpful Tools for Professionals Use in Fighting the Opioid Epidemic

State Prescription Drug Monitoring Program (SPDMP)

The creation of a computerized prescription database that collects data on prescriptions written and dispensed and making them available for physicians/ providers have helped immensely in this opioid epidemic.[1]

The SPDMP is a state-provided computerized database which goes by many different names or acronyms, depending on each particular state. Data are usually kept and made available for about one year for each prescription written for each patient that contains any drug classified Schedule II – V. It also lists the pharmacies and the date(s) that each prescription was filled by the pharmacy, which may be the same date the patient picked up the medications.

However, sometimes the patients may pick up their medications after the filled dates, usually within a few days, or most pharmacies will call them if they failed to pick up their filled medications in a timely manner.

The database also contains most of the relevant information from the patient's prescription. There is also a summary which lists the total number of pharmacies, total number of prescribers, the number of prescriptions, and the number of opioids/ control substances and their **MME daily dose** for that particular patient. Each pharmacy and provider's contact information/addresses are also listed. Generally, the information available in the different states' database is similar but varies from state to state.

It is generally about 95%-plus accurate; inaccuracies are sometimes seen in the patient's name, address, the date the prescription was written, the date the prescription was filled, date of birth, the number of pills dispensed, and the prescribing doctors. However, these inaccuracies can often be resolved with a phone call to the pharmacy and a review of the patient's medical records, among other things. The benefits of SPDMP are significant; most of us can tolerate a few glitches for the number of benefits we get.

Trends and plans are on the way to make these databases regional, with the goal of eventually being national. This will require states wherein the programs are now voluntary in operation to become mandatory. Adding to this will be the need for the immediate reporting of data entry for each prescription as it is dispensed. There are states/pharmacies in which the entry of data into the system takes a few days and even longer, thereby allowing the possibility of **doctor-shopping** within that time frame. There are, of course, additional costs that must be absorbed by pharmacies which have the potential to make smaller pharmacies less compliant partly because of the additional financial burden required to operate and maintain the database. Currently, the SPDMP is not available in every state and/or not utilized by all pharmacies. Also, the information required for the database from some emergency rooms /urgent care centers, methadone clinics and nursing homes or skilled nursing facilities that are dispensing or filling prescriptions are sometimes not captured in a significant number of states. Additionally, the information in some of them is poorly recorded. However, with the current opioid epidemic, monitoring and new protocols in place in emergency rooms and urgent care centers are prescribing less and fewer opioids or controlled substances. Once a system/program becomes more truly national, this will have a significant impact on identifying patients who are trying to obtain multiple prescriptions and have them filled (doctor-shopping).

Also, as the opioid epidemic expands or as we try to get better control of this crisis, more medications are likely to be added to the drugs schedule as the potential for their abuse becomes more apparent. For example, gabapentin, a non-opioid drug, is now considered a drug with significant abuse potential. It may conceivably be upgraded to Schedule V and be a part of the SPDMP in the near future, as pregabalin currently is.

The state of Georgia's PDMP allows providers to see prescriptions given by providers in Georgia, South Carolina, Alabama, Massachusetts, Mississippi, and North Dakota by the end of May 2018. Currently, at the end of October 2018, the number was up to fifteen as others state are being added to the database, this is a work in progress.

I called the administering agency for the Georgia PDMP on June 4, 2018. The most I could take from what was said is that the process is evolving, and some states are just not in a position at this time to share data, and others may be unwilling to share. However, the process is getting better in light of the opioid epidemic.

Some states are requiring that providers writing opioids and other controlled substances must check their state database before giving prescriptions to new patients. The databases may also provide additional alerts for providers who are seeing patients who have multiple prescribers or drugs that they are prescribed and do not fit the normally expected pattern.[1]

However, once up and fully running in all states, when patients from whichever part of the country walk into a medical provider's office, that provider will at least have that patient's prescription history for about a year. So, if you are a consumer reading this book and I trust that your intentions are good, please advise anyone that you may know that not only is it illegal to obtain multiple opioid prescriptions from different doctors but also they will be caught.

Urine Drug Testing (UDT)

UDT is one of the most important tools available to help in the fight against the opioid epidemic. For most reputable pain management practices, UDT remains one of the single most objective diagnostic tests available for therapeutic monitoring, compliance, and determining patients' use of medications/illicit drugs, among other things. However, UDT is not without its share of problems and controversies.[2]

In most instances UDT constitutes what are referred to as **presumptive** or **qualitative testing**, and **definitive testing** also called **quantitative testing** or **confirmation testing**. In presumptive testing, we most commonly see what is called **Point-of-Care Testing (POCT)** and **Immunoassay (IA)** or **Chemistry Analyzer Testing**.

In **POCT,** the patients' urine samples may be collected in diagnostic specimen cups that have a specimen grid that allows visual interpretations of different substances in the sample. Similarly, the urine may be collected; and dipsticks/ strips, cassettes or specimen cards with grids are used to test and visually interpret samples with respect to the substances or compounds contained. Although the results are very basic, they are immediately obtainable and can often be used to make decisions about the treatment of patients on opioids, other controlled substances or illegal drugs.

It is very useful at times and is the more frequently used test outside of pain management practices (as well as some pain management practices). Most primary care offices and family practice offices rely on this form of testing to a significant degree. But these tests have very high risks of false-positive and false-negative results. Therefore, their use as primary determinants to manage patients are very risky, to say the least.

The next **presumptive or qualitative test** is performed by a machine referred to as a **chemistry analyzer**; the test is an **IA test**. Patients' samples are collected and tested using machines which have been validated for testing specific substances or compounds. This process is significantly more rigorous than a POCT. These results can be obtained in a few hours. However, because of the logistics of the process, the expected time depends on many factors, such as where the testing is done (whether on-site at the physician's office or reference labs), and the available personnel, among others. The results may be available the next day or longer, unlike those of POCT. The results from these tests are generally reported as positive or negative, indicating the presence or absence of drugs or drug classes, or in some instances, specific drugs may be identified in a given urine sample.

Definitive, quantitative or confirmation testing is also necessary to confirm or validate the results of tests that were done presumptively if indicated. The instruments commonly used are a combined machine consisting of **chromatography and mass spectrometry**. In most instances, **liquid chromatography** is used. However, the less popular and less accurate **gas chromatography** may also be used. The machines are also required to undergo an extensive validation process that is directly related to the specimens and/or compounds that will be tested.

The time frame for the validation process will depend on many factors, some of which are personnel, the compounds being validated for testing, and the type of machines and their manufacturer. This typically takes weeks, whereas the analyser – IA validation may take about a week, depending on many factors as well.[2]

These definitive or confirmation tests are done to identify or confirm specific medications, illicit drugs, and metabolites of substances consumed. These results are reported indicating the presence or absence of substances in their specific concentration, usually in units of nanograms per milliliter (ng/ml). The results of definitive/confirmation testing are extremely accurate.

Not every sample that is presumptively tested requires confirmation testing. The need for confirmation is dictated by many factors such as the results of the presumptive tests, expectations of results based on patient history, the medications the patient is currently taking and how that reconciles with the results.

The turnaround time for these results may vary significantly, depending on where the definitive testing is done. In some of the more established pain management practices that are also physician-owned laboratories, the turnaround time varies but may be done in a few days. Sometimes these are sent to be tested at reference laboratories and have a similar time frame for returning results.

Presumptive UDT, POCT or chemistry analyzer or IA testing, as well as definitive or confirmation testing, require compliance and approval by the state and Centers for Medicare and Medicaid Services (CMS). "**The Clinical Laboratory Improvement Amendments (CLIA)** regulates laboratory testing and requires clinical labs to be certified by their state as well as CMS before they can accept human samples for diagnostic testing." CLIA will issue certification depending on the level of complexity of testing and requirements met by each provider performing tests. This may be minimal (Wave), moderate or complex laboratory certification.

The laboratory may have been established in a physician's office (physician-owned); or may be separate from the office, owned by non-physicians or business owners, often called or functioning as a **reference lab.** All laboratories, whether **physician- owned** or reference lab, must meet the same requirement for special certifications and compliance adherence to operating.

As mentioned earlier, reliance on presumptive testing, which identifies the presence or absence of drugs or drug classes, or in some instances, substances or specific drugs, is both very useful and very risky. The reason for this is the poor sensitivity and cross-reactivity which limit the accuracy and reliability of the tests. Therefore, the negative test results do not always indicate the absence of compounds in the urine sample; and neither do positive results necessarily tell us what substances are actually present, as we may be looking at a class of drugs rather than a specific positive drug.

This may become extremely important, particularly when managing patients who are using controlled substances/opioids, illegal drugs or other substances that may exacerbate the difficulties of managing their cases.

Definitive or confirmation testing also has limitations, of course. It cannot and is not used to test and identify every substance there is, or probably may be present. The test is not required to do this for them to be effective. Also, as mentioned before, not every compound that is negative or positive that is being presumptively tested requires the need for confirmation.[2] In spite of the sensitivity, specificity, or simply the accuracy of this, there are still many substances that will go undetected for numerous reasons.

All definitive or confirmation testing labs can only validate and perform specific tests for a limited number of substances and/or their metabolites. There are numerous analogs/designer drugs that will be missed on testing. The cost of these tests is very expensive because of the nature and complexity involved in performing accurate testing, as well as the personnel required for appropriate results analysis and interpretation, and maintaining compliance with regulatory bodies. There are other factors and limitations of definitive or confirmation testing as well.

Other Types of Monitoring of Opioids and Controlled Substances

Oral swabs: For patients who are unable to void or produce urine, an oral swab is often used to determine similar information available from the urine sample. These samples are frequently collected and sent to reference labs for analysis and confirmation. It is also equally useful in helping manage patients in a pain management setting who are using opioids and other controlled substances and are unable to avoid them. The results from the testing have a turnaround time comparable to confirmation testing.

Genetic Testing

Genetic testing is also referred to as **pharmacogenomics**. It is for patients who are using opioid medications, and other controlled substances is gradually becoming more popular. The concept has to do with the fact that all patients metabolizing the substances or compounds that they ingest do so differently, to some degree. In theory, our genomes determine how we metabolize products. Some patients are seen in medical practices and found to respond poorly to some medications while responding well to others.

There are also some patients who can tolerate a very large dose of opioids/ other substances, while others are unable to do so. This may be in part due to some patients being able to metabolize substances/medications much faster than others for the same comparable period, age range and medical condition. In general, patients who are fast metabolizers will tolerate large doses of medication unlike those who are slow metabolizers of comparable ages and medical status.

This question always arises: how much of these phenomena in each patient have anything to do with their genetic makeup or genome?

One of the hopes is that genetic testing in individual patients will allow healthcare providers/physicians to have or create a more customized treatment approach for each patient with respect to their needs for opioids or other medications, based on their genetic makeup. Although genetic testing can and will play an important role in customizing patients' medication treatment, the science is still evolving.

Genetic testing is not only useful in opioid treatment. It has also found use in possibly customizing medication treatment protocols for a wide range of other known medical conditions where different medications are available for use in treating similar or the same conditions, but different patients respond differently. Of course, if genetic testing results can dictate with greater accuracy each patient's needs for opioids/other controlled substances and medications as a whole, we would have another formidable opponent against the opioid epidemic.

The establishment of a laboratory that performs genetic testing also has to adhere to regulatory compliance as well as obtain the appropriate certifications required to operate similarly to the other testing labs described above.

Specimen Validity Testing

The collection of urine samples in the hands of most patients will not be tampered with or subjected to any alteration that will change the testing outcomes. Unfortunately, there is a significant number of patients who have chosen to add various compounds or other substances to the urine specimens in order to obtain a specific result or to mask other substances such as illegal drugs that may be in the urine. Validity testing, which includes but are not limited to **specific gravity**, **pH**, **oxidants**, and **creatinine** is very useful.

These tests ensure that the urine samples that are collected and subjected to presumptive testing are appropriate, and has decreased risks of contaminants or adulterants. These tests may be performed presumptively using the chemistry analyzer. They are not typically done with POCT. As important as they are, most healthcare insurance companies do not pay for them.

Problems of and Controversies Regarding UDT

How do we determine when and how many times to test patients who are using opioids chronically and are being monitored or under the care of a pain management practice? Presently, we also have to ask, how does this help in fighting the opioid epidemic?

Medicare has established a guideline for treatment as well as frequencies. However, this is intended to be a guideline, and patient management is supposed to be determined by the physicians and/or medical providers.[4]

Over the years, we've seen many large testing companies involved in litigations resulting in the refund of large sums of money to healthcare insurance companies, including governmental insurance such as Medicare and Medicaid. Medical doctors and/or healthcare providers have also been involved in cases where the refund of large sums of money for what was considered unnecessary testing was among some of the indicated reasons. In addition, there are a significant number of healthcare insurance companies that have found it convenient and justifiable to deny a large number of legitimate claims for completed UDT. This is generally easy because there is no set policy or protocol which is considered the standard of care to be followed.

Therefore, each healthcare insurance company sets its own policies and protocols on how UDT should be done. And at any time of the year, they can and often do change their implemented policies and protocols. Of course, the policies, protocols, and guidelines that they write are sometimes not consistent with the scientific basis of UDT or have very little to do with the management of patients being treated.

However, these protocols or policy guidelines are often based on how much financial exposure or liability each healthcare insurance company is willing to accept. The needs of the patients are generally not taken into consideration in most cases. Similarly, healthcare providers and their ability to adequately manage their patients' opioid use are secondary to the financial needs of most healthcare insurance companies.

How Often Should Physicians/Providers Perform UDT for the Patients who were Prescribed Opioids for Chronic Pain?

The CDC guidelines suggest the following:

When prescribing opioids for chronic pain, clinicians should use urine drug testing before starting opioid therapy and consider urine drug testing at least annually to assess for prescribed medications as well as other controlled prescription drugs and illicit drugs.[3]

So, after the first testing, that should be followed by (at least) annual testing. Now let's assume that patient John or Mary had their first test and there was no issue at all; clean as a whistle, as they say.

Now you see this patient over the next 11 months; when do we test again? How often and why? This should be guided in part by the medical needs and the risk of the patient concerning the use of opioids and other controlled substances, among many other things.

Here are some general thoughts: a significant number of patients coming to pain management for opioids with the potential risk of abuse are more likely to present themselves as clean or free from illegal drugs and, if possible, present medical record of compliance with respect to legal drugs.

What happens in the months that follow is anybody's guess. Once the patient feels that no monitoring is in place, they often default to their normal mode of operation. In most practices, the patients who will be caught doing illegal activities, misusing or abusing opioids or controlled substances are those who are subjected to consecutive screenings that are not necessarily predictable. Doing predictable monthly or every-three-months UDT may not necessarily result in the abnormal findings that will lead to information necessary to discharge patients or to take corrective actions. If the patients present to a clinic every three months and obtain a UDT at each time, that often does not lead to results that are useful, unlike tests that are randomly done and less predictable for patients. The same applies to any monthly tests that are done routinely. What generally yield very reliable and meaningful results are tests performed on them that are generally non-predictable. This allows for patients to be tested consecutively or be called in for a random drug test as the medical need dictates. Most patients discharged from practices are usually discharged because they are often caught essentially unprepared for UDT. Then you find the "good patients" with some amazing stuff from illegal drugs to undisclosed control substances, misuse of opioids and others.

A similar scenario applies to medications review or pills count, where patients' chance of predicting is less likely, and a more realistic review or count can be accomplished.

Medications Review – Pills Count

Medications review is the process of having patients present to their providers' office on short notice and without prior knowledge of this appointment. They are required to bring all their medications prescribed to them by all the doctors/ providers treating them, in their respective containers. This is often done to reconcile patients' medical history and dispensed prescriptions.

This also gives us a chance to determine the need for patients' medications adequacy and make appropriate adjustments. Patients are generally discharged if they fail to attend or show up for these appointments without a substantially good and verifiable reason.

Sometimes, patients may show up with almost all or some of the prescriptions mixed up in one container, or some of the medications are not found in the original prescribed container. In some instances, patients may even have medications in containers that are different than what they were prescribed in, but rather in containers that are old and have different medications that were given in the past. Understanding the rationale for patients' storage of medications or lack thereof can be helpful in determining their risks for diversion, as well as compliance in taking all their medications as prescribed.

Failure to demonstrate satisfactorily appropriate use of prescribed medications opioids/controlled substances generally lead to immediate discharge. Some patients, probably knowing that they are abusing are misusing medications, may simply have failed, and don't show up and are discharged. Some of the more blatant ones will try to substitute or show different medications than what was prescribed. However, whatever tricks that are used by noncompliant patients, medications reviews are extremely important in helping in the fight against the opioid epidemic.

Local Pharmacy Monitoring – Fake Prescriptions and More

Local pharmacies also play key roles in helping the opioid epidemics. Most of these pharmacies will know the practices that are around, and the prescriptions that most of the providers are likely to write. Some of them will be familiar with even the signatures of some of the providers. They are the gatekeepers of fake prescriptions that have increased in numbers over the last few years. It is easy for anyone to obtain physicians' national provider identifier (NPI), license and or DEA numbers. There are individuals who have spent much time writing prescriptions using providers' credentials for opioids/controlled substances and do get them filled.

It is so important to keep the doors of communication open between providers and pharmacists. It is great when your local pharmacists can call and verify or intercept prescriptions that may have been created by a fraudulent person, or intercept and stop a prescription that has fallen into the wrong hands from being dispensed.

More recently, pharmacists are paying closer attention to IDs and even to the addresses of the patients on the prescriptions. Some pharmacists are now even calling to verify not only the identity of the person whom the prescription was prescribed to but also to verify the correct address of the patients.

Law enforcement also plays a role in helping to bring to justice the perpetrators of fraudulent opioid-prescription crimes.

Local pharmacists also play a role in reporting what is considered abnormal prescriptions: this may include the quantity of opioids/controlled substances to be dispensed, the type of medications, the frequency of medications or anything that is considered outside the norm of their pharmaceutical judgment. Providers/ Prescribers are sometimes reported to various regulatory bodies including the State Medical Boards and the DEA, among others. Some pharmacists will be kind enough to put in personal phone calls directly to the provider's office to verify or confirm what they considered outside of the normal boundaries of prescriptions. These calls are almost always helpful; and provide additional layers of protection to all the parties involved; the patients, pharmacists, and providers/prescribers.

With the opioid epidemic continuing and with no apparent end in sight, sometimes in an effort to be cautious or safe, some pharmacists tend to make calls that at times may seem to be more of a knee-jerk reaction or failure to understand the full context in which the call is made. For example, there are times when pain management offices, as well as the prescribers of the controlled medication in question, will be called because a patient is on opioids and a benzo, even for small doses such as hydrocodone 5/325 mg and Xanax 0.25 mg once daily.

The questions often asked by the pharmacists: are you aware of the medications the patient is taken and the danger he or she is in? Now although this may be considered irritating by some providers, the principle behind the call is solid. Indeed, this is one last and very important step some pharmacists are required to take which can often help to protect both providers as well as our patients.

Large Pharmacies' Database Prescription Review

Most physicians/medical providers that have been practicing even for a short period will have patients who are prescribed a large number of different medications from different providers. They will sometimes have different providers that prescribe similar or sometimes the same medications that they are getting from other providers who are also treating them.

Some of these issues can be resolved with a good medical history from the patients, or sometimes electronic medical records. There is now an electronic interface or a device connected with some patients' prescription–pharmacy database, which allow the providers to see prescriptions that they are not providing.

The larger private health insurance companies, governmental or state health insurance companies have pharmaceutical divisions that have a computerized database of most, if not all, of the medications prescribed to each of their patients.

The healthcare insurance companies and their associates are able to conduct **drug utilization reviews** in an effort to provide educational information, promote safety, and provide or facilitate the appropriate use of medications for their patients.

They often send out correspondences about patients who fall in the categories that they deem appropriate for review. These reviews may take the form of simple questionnaires to be completed by the providers regarding patients' use of one or more medications. These may be, among other things: possible drugs interactions, age appropriateness concerning certain medications, patients on medications that are essentially similar from one or more different providers, the doses of medications, and questions or information about the possible worsening of certain medical conditions. Examples of some of those companies are **Optum Rx**, **Caremark**, and **Silverscript**.

For Concerned Consumers and Patients

The enormity of the problem caused by the opioid epidemic cannot be overemphasized. I have mentioned several times in this book that this problem requires all of us to be participants in finding solutions. At some point in our lives, this will reach us or our family members or friends.

It is always welcoming to see concerned citizens and patients who decided to be a part of the solution rather than sit on the side lines and wait to see what will happen next. In simple terms:

"if you see something, say something."

I have provided a list of websites and phone numbers at the end of this book. Feel free to utilize them; you'll find them to be great resources.

Not-so-Useful Tool; Opioid
Pre-Authorization from Healthcare Insurances

The pre-authorization from healthcare insurance companies for opioid use for longer than seven days by pain management physicians/providers does very little, if anything, to help with reversing, controlling, or making any significant impact on the opioid epidemic. Although this is a protocol that is recently implemented for opioids, and there are no significant data available to show its impact at this time, it is highly probably that in the long run, no significant gain will be achieved.

Pre-authorization has always been a challenge for pain management practices over the years, however, medications that often require preauthorization are medications that would be very helpful in providing alternatives for opioids or better opioids in treating chronic pain.

These medications include but are not limited to non-opioids and opioids-deterrent formulations. Healthcare insurance companies often don't approve a significant number of these medications.

A considerable amount of time is consumed in obtaining pre-authorization for patients who have been on opioids beforehand and may have stopped for a brief period, and then resumed taking them. Office staff/providers have to complete multiple forms and or sometimes spend more than thirty minutes for each medication or patient on the phone with healthcare insurance representatives to obtain pre-authorization for the opioid medications prescribed, creating more of a hassle for both patients and their providers rather than a solution to a greater problem.

Depending on the state that you are practicing a healthcare insurance company or a regulatory body will tell you that you cannot prescribe more than 3 to 7 days of opioids for acute pain for someone who is being "started" on an opioid medication. In some instance, if the patient was using opioids chronically but stop for more than 30 or 60 days then that patient is should be considered as if he or she is a new patient being treated for the first time. This applies even if he or she has been taking opioids but failed to fill a prescription for opioid for more than 30 or 60 days depending on the insurance or regulatory body.

CMS has a publication from Medicare Learning Network (#SE 18016) titled "**A Prescriber's Guide to New Medicare Part D Opioid Overutilization Policies for 2019**".

This publication also indicates that CMS will have a requirement of "seven- day supply limit" for opioid-naive patients who have the need to be started on opioids. This publication, however, has other important guidelines the will be or expected to be implemented in 2019 and will affect both providers and patients. Two examples from this publication are; Pharmacy Limitation also known as "pharmacy lock in" and Prescriber Limitation known as "prescriber lock in."[5]

References, Recommended Readings and Resources

1. The Centers for Disease Control and Prevention. CDC. What States Need to Know about PDMPs. https://www.cdc.gov/drugoverdose/ pdmp/states. html. Last visited July 13, 2018.
2. Local Coverage Determination (LCD): Controlled Substance Monitoring and Drugs of Abuse Testing (L36393). Centers for Medicare and Medicaid Services.LastrevisedJanuary17, 2018.https://www.cms.gov/medicare-cov- erage-database/details/lcd- details.aspx?LC- DId=36393&ver=24&Do-cID=L36393&bc=iAAAABAAAAAA&. Accessed on July 31, 2018.
3. Deborah Dowell, MD; Tamara M. Haegerich, Ph.D.; Roger Chou, MD. CDC Guideline for Prescribing Opioids for Chronic Pain. Morbidity and Mortality Weekly Report (MMWR). March 18, 2016. https://www.cdc.gov/ mmwr/volumes/65/rr/rr6501e1.htm. Accessed July 23, 2018.
4. Matthew J. Bair MD, MS Erin E. Krebs MD, MPH. Why Is Urine Drug Testing Not Used More Often in Practice? 29 October 2010. Pain Prac- tice. November/December 2010: 10(6): 493 – 496. https:// onlinelibrary. wiley.com/doi/full/10.1111/j.1533-2500.2010.00425.x. Last visited July 23, 2018.
5. A Prescriber's Guide to the New Medicare Part D Opioid Overutilization Policies for 2019. https://www.cms.gov/Outreach- and-Education/Medi- care-Learning-Network-MLN/MLNMattersArticles/Downloads/SE18016. pdf Last visited November 29, 2018.

Chapter 15

What are the Pharmaceutical Companies Doing?

The pharmaceutical industry, medical providers/doctors, and politicians/ government are considered to have played the central role in the opioid epidemic. In the early 1990s until about the year 2010 prescription opioids gradually increased to a maximum. Over that period, it essentially quadrupled. The deaths from opioid overdose increased by fivefold from 1999 to 2016.[1,4]

OxyContin, oxycodone, hydrocodone, fentanyl, and morphine are some of the opioids that saw a significant increase in sales and demand. OxyContin or oxycodone was one of the most marketed opioids; the marketing campaign involved print media as well as commercials and infomercials.

Medical providers/prescribers were specifically marketed to and were sometimes given things of value. This had the potential for inducement, with the intention of writing more prescriptions for their products. In addition, although opioids were intended for palliative care and end-of-life/cancer care treatment, products like OxyContin became more and more popular for the treatment of general chronic pain that was noncancer-related.[2,3] There was also the promotion of opioids not being significantly addictive.

The addictive potential of opioids was simply minimized, and the potential benefits for pain management were emphasized, not only by the pharmaceutical companies but also by significant members of the medical community as well as several medical associations.

There have been many lawsuits against the pharmaceutical industry, brought forward by different states and their municipalities as well as individuals. Several representatives and/or executives have been arrested and charged with crimes in the pharmaceutical industry. Some of them pleaded guilty, and there are still ongoing litigations.

In an effort to decrease the risks of misuse and abuse, some pharmaceutical companies have manufactured what is referred to as abuse-deterrent drugs. Some of the more common ones that are FDA-approved are **Hysingla ER**, **Embeda**, **Morphabond ER**, **Xtampza ER**, **Arymo ER**, and **OxyContin**. The idea behind these medications is to make it more difficult for patients to abuse them, or use them in ways different from how they were intended to be used. These are long-acting or extended-release opioids which are currently available. The FDA has also approved an immediate release opioid with abuse-deterrent formulation property called **RoxyBond** (Oxycodone). It is the first FDA short- acting abuse- deterrent formulation opioid; this is expected to be available for prescription about January 2019.

The cost of these medications is generally higher than conventional medications of similar types. A significant number of patients often are not able to benefit from them because of their costs. Also, most medical health insurance will not pay for them, or if they do, they will pay for only one or maybe two of those on rare occasions on their available formulary lists. However, the patients who do try to fill these prescriptions sometimes have very high coinsurance or co-pays, resulting in most patients being unable to purchase these medications, even with their health insurance.

Another factor that often arises from this is that some patients who were not able to obtain the more expensive formulations will sometime resort to illegal drugs (such as heroin or IMF) if the regular, cheaper medications are not readily available or if they are no longer prescribed to them. Another compounding factor is that heroin and IMF are usually much cheaper than the conventional or generic non- deterrent formulation.

Among the many questions that must be asked are: are the prices of prescription drugs fair and reasonable? In other words, are pharmaceutical companies selling their products at fair prices to the consumers? If the prices are not fair and reasonable, then that will make it less likely that most of these drugs will be purchased or covered by health insurance companies. Which of course will lead to the situation we currently have, where medications are available, but only a few people who can afford them or will benefit from them.

I'm not in the least saying or implying that pharmaceutical companies should not profit. After all, the process of manufacturing drugs and getting them ready to be marketed to consumers with FDA approval is not an easy or cheap process. It is not uncommon that during the development or manufacturing of these new or potential drugs that there are many failed attempts before the final products are realized.

However, there has to be a balance that facilitates more reasonable prices for drugs and better coverage of medications so that more people can have a meaningful chance of receiving those drugs. Having access to the medications you want but not being able to afford them simply makes it useless.

Of course, the same thing applies to healthcare insurance in general; we all have access possibly to the greatest medical care available in the world right here in the United States, but yet so many are unable to afford or receive it. So what good does it do for those who cannot afford it?

The role of politicians has not gone unnoticed; some of them simply acquiesced to the source of largest monetary contributions or strongest lobbying force. Many of the members of the Congress and Senate have long been influenced by donations from both the pharmaceutical and healthcare insurance companies, as well as other companies. Many of these sectors have significant lobbying arms that are committed to making sure that the interests of their industry are addressed. Unfortunately, in some instances, the interests and goals of specific companies may not necessarily be of benefit to or be reconciled with the needs of the consumers or the people who are at the greatest risk. Unfortunately, lobbying and big donations to various politicians that ultimately have a significant impact on legislation seem likely to stay.

This is not something that is unique to one political party or specific industry or group of politicians. This is common throughout our political system, and with the exception of a few minor and occasional changes, in all probability things will remain the same.

The level of marketing that is believed to have contributed to the driving force behind the increased availability of prescriptions is, apparently, significantly less than it used to be. The number of constant and frequent commercials for opioid use is down. Also, pharmaceutical representatives who often visit healthcare providers' offices are being seen less and less. In February 2018, a letter was sent out to providers' offices from a major pharmaceutical company stating that the company will no longer be visiting providers' offices and engaging in discussions about the opioid products that it sells. However, moving forward, the correspondence stated, direct communication with their specialized staff will handle questions and requests for information about their opioid products.

References, Recommended Readings and Resources

1. Centers for Disease Control and Prevention. Understanding the Epidemic. https://www.cdc.gov/drugoverdose/epidemic/index.html. Last visited June 16, 2018.

2. Sean Adl-Tabatabai. Harvard Study: Big Pharma, US Gov. Behind Opioid Epidemic. July 27, 2017, News, US 105. https://yournewswire. com/harvard-study-opioid-epidemic/. Accessed March 12,2018.

3. Ritchie Farrell. The Opioid Epidemic: How Big Pharma and Congress Created America's Worst Health Crisis. 10/16/2017. https://www. huffington-post.com/entry/the-opioid-epidemic-how-big-pharma-and- congress-created_us_59e4e02ee4b003f928d5e8bf. Accessed March7, 2018

4. Gery P. Guy Jr., Ph.D.; Kun Zhang, Ph.D.; Michele K. Bohm, MPH; Jan Losby, Ph.D.; Brian Lewis; Randall Young, MA; Louise B. Murphy, Ph.D.; Deborah Dowell, MD· CDCMMWR. Vital Signs: Changes in Opioid Pre- scribing in the United States, 2006–2015. July 7, 2017 / 66(26);697- 704. https://www.cdc.gov/mmwr/volumes/66/wr/ mm6626a4.htm?s_cid=m- m6626a4_w. Accessed March 1,2018.

Chapter 16

What are the Federal and State Government Doing?

The Challenges

The opioid epidemic is one of immense magnitude. The effect of the epidemic has not gone unnoticed by the federal or state government. The influence of the federal government is significant. Numerous agencies have a direct impact on the epidemic through research, education, funding projects, public awareness campaigns, legislation, community activism, and others. Part of the challenge is trying to keep up with a very complex problem that has many moving parts. Although the problem itself is not new, the scale and magnitude have definitely surpassed the usual measures to contain it. Addiction to drugs such as crack cocaine and heroin have been with us for several decades.

However, the opioid epidemic has taken on a new level of crisis, with deaths now quadrupled from what they used to be 20 to 30 years ago. We watch our emergency services, medical facilities, and personnel being overloaded. We see hospitals and medical facilities increasing their resources trying to catch up with an escalating crisis, but still falling short at times.

The budgets for healthcare, law enforcement, and related services have ballooned out of proportion to what had been customary. There is no doubt that more money is needed to be put into the system to address the opioid epidemic and all the different sectors and factors that are affected financially.

The opioid epidemic overall is looked at as driven by the overprescription of legal opioids. This escalation began in the late 1990s and continued to increase to a maximum level to about 2010, which is when legal prescriptions over that period quadrupled.[1,2]

The second factor that has contributed to the epidemic is the increased availability of illegal opioids such as heroin and IMF. The demand for illicit opioids increased dramatically as the supply from legally prescribed opioids decreased, and there was a larger number of opioid users and addicted patients partly because of the decrease in diversion opioids.

The third factor was that illegally manufactured opioids such as fentanyl and heroin became much cheaper, more potent and more readily available. Added to this, designer or analog drugs increased in supply and availability; and decreased in price.[3]

Crackdown on Pill mills

Among some of the measures taken by states was a crackdown on Pill mills. This had the effect of removing a significant amount of opioid diversions that were "legally prescribed," as well as the so-called "pain doctors" and businesspeople who were profiting illegally and unethically from these clinics. The concept of Pill mills seems to have evolved and grown in parallel with the increase in pain prescriptions for opioids from about the year 2000, and become more significant in about 2010.[1]

The laws and rules that banned their activities of prescribing opioids illegally and primarily for profit are often referred to as the Pill mill Laws. Many states have adopted similar laws to govern the operations of pain clinics. Although there are differences between the various states' laws, there are certain features held in common by these laws. These may include: the clinic must be owned by a physician who is licensed or trained in the practice of pain medicine or appropriately credentialed, therefore eliminating the businessman who typically funds these clinics and uses often retired or semi-retired physicians simply to write prescriptions. These clinics would be limited to dispensing opioids and other controlled substances from their office unless they are registered with their State's Pharmacy Board or State Medical Board.

The law also requires that clinics that treat more than 50% of its patients as pain management patients with Schedule II-III controlled substances/narcotics must be registered, and part of its name must be reflected to include "pain" in the name of the practice. In addition, these patients must be properly assessed and evaluated to determine if they are appropriate for pain management treatment prior to the start of treatment and monitored properly during treatment.

Failure to comply with the law may lead to a felony conviction; no one with a felony conviction would be granted a license to operate or own a pain clinic.

The Comparative Billing Report Program

The CMS has a program that is administered through a third-party provider that looks at how providers bill procedures and/or office visits or ancillary services. If the providers fall outside of the range of what is considered normal, then they may receive a notification from the third-party provider regarding their method of practice or billing.

For example, if a vascular surgeon performed significantly more lower limb amputations than other providers in the same specialty over the same period, then there's a possibility that the surgeon would be considered outside of the norm of practice. Similarly, for the opioid prescribers and pain management practices/ providers, the program also monitors how opioids are prescribed to Medicare Part D beneficiaries.

The program looks at the following categories:

➢ The number of prescriptions written
➢ Total number of beneficiaries
➢ The average charge by pharmacies for medications prescribed by prescribers.
➢ The percentage of the prescribers' patients receiving more
➢ than 90 MME daily dose of opioids
➢ The average number of days of each prescription is written for each beneficiary
➢ The percentage of beneficiaries which the prescriber prescribed that has seen four or more providers.

These categories are looked at generally for a period of 12 months. The providers are then compared to each other in the specialty of pain management. Also, each provider in pain management is compared with all other specialties combined nationally. The non-providers of pain management are compared to the nationally combined specialties, as well as to the specialty of pain management. Each provider can then examine his or her data average with respect to opioid prescriptions for the categories listed above, and determine where corrective measures might be helpful. The average for each category in each specialty is then compared to each provider's pattern of opioid prescription.

The program appears to focus on getting providers to be aware of how they are prescribing opioids or their prescription patterns, and possibly make appropriate adjustments. This program does not consider each practice's unique or varying patient population or the specific regional area the providers are located. There is no medical record utilized other than the pure data ascertained from the prescriptions dispensed database.

The 90 MME is significant and is in keeping with most of the established guidelines such as the CDC's. The average cost per prescription may shed some light on the possibility of those whose cost per prescription may indicate possible inducements or preference for particular drugs that may be more expensive, among other things. The average number of days' prescriptions will vary from practice to practice and may reflect the nature and type of practice that providers are a part of. Looking at patients who have had multiple prescriptions from multiple providers over one year does not give necessarily a true reflection of the provider's failure to monitor their patients who are using multiple prescribers or are doctor- shopping.

Among the reasons for this is that although multiple doctors may be in the same practices, they are still counted as different doctors/providers. Also, if a patient is seen in your office today and you prescribed one prescription for opioids and never see that patient again, that patient has about 11 months or so to receive opioids from three or more doctors, whether it be from the emergency room, dentists, primary care, or other physicians. I have had discussions with a representative at CMS; the program is still evolving, with the future possibility of providers having access to their information for prescribing as the data are collected and recorded.[8]

The DEA Sets Quota to Reduce the Production of Schedule II Opioids

The DEA determine the amount of medication that various pharmaceutical companies produce each year in the United States. It does this by examining and analyzing sales data, and the usage and surplus of medications, among other factors. It proposed what is called an Aggregate Production Quota (APQ) for each class and/or type of drugs or compounds.[4,5,6,32] This topic is covered in chapter 5 of this book.

According to a recent article by CNN, the overall reduction in opioid production has resulted in surgical procedures in some hospitals being significantly hampered because of the inadequate amounts of intravenous opioids such as Morphine, Dilaudid and fentanyl.[7]

The CMS has Proposed Limits to be Enacted for Opioid Prescriptions

The CMS has proposed in April 2018 limits to be enacted for prescriptions in the guidelines for patients receiving their insurance through CMS (Medicare Part D). The maximum amount of opioids that will be allowed to be dispensed will be **90 MME** per day or daily.[9] The MME per day, also referred to as the **Morphine Equivalent Dose (MED)** per day, is a fundamental terminology or concept in opioid treatment.

Every provider who prescribes opioids needs to understand its significance and how it is calculated. There is also a benefit to consumers who are inclined to be more involved in their treatment to know what their MMEs are. MME calculations use morphine as the reference opioid base on the strength or potency of other opioids.

The CDC has a conversion table which is available for use. Although it does not cover some opioids, it still forms a significant reference point from which to determine the MME of each patient who is prescribed opioids. The table and the conversion factors are shown in Appendix A[10]

In general, 90 MME/day equates to each patient having a maximum allowable daily dose of about: morphine 90 mg (example, three tablets of morphine 30 mg), hydrocodone 90 mg (nine tablets of hydrocodone 10/325), oxycodone 60 mg (four tablets of oxycodone 15 mg), or methadone 20 mg (four tablets of methadone 5 mg). Any combination of pills and/or medications, in general, is allowable for each day of 90 MME/day.[10] The supply would be initially limited to seven days for acute pain. This is expected to be effective in 2019. This limit is also consistent with the CDC guidelines of 2016 for primary care providers. The question of course remains: will this at some point in time be extended or be enacted for chronic pain patients?[9,11]

As a consumer, you may look at this and say, "Good! Now I can have adequate pain control." That is correct, but don't expect to go to your primary care doctors or your pain management doctors/providers and expect to receive the full amount of 90 MME per day of opioids. In facts, rarely any or very few patients will ever receive this amount of opioids for initial treatments. This equivalent quantity of opioids is a significant amount even for the vast majority of chronic pain patients. Referring to data from the Comparative Billing Report Program for the period of July 1, 2016 to June 30, 2017 for Medicare Part D patients, only 4% nationally from all other providers/doctors were prescribed 90 MME per day or more of opioids; while from pain management specialists, 14% of patients received 90 MME/day or more of opioids. Overall, it is a good thing that a more significant number of patients is not receiving a considerable amount of opioids.

Statistics have consistently shown that there are increased risks of overdose that correlate with the increasing amounts of opioids that patients take. A national sample of the Veterans Health Administration or VHA of chronic pain patients revealed that patients who have overdosed were found to have an average of 98 MME/day (more deaths), while those with 50 MME/day were associated with fewer deaths. However, there is an increased risk of doubling the potential overdose for patients receiving more than 50 MME/day compared to patients with doses that are less than 20 MME/day.[10]

Some States are Passing New Laws or Implementing New Rules

Some states like New York now require mandatory prescription-education courses in order to be qualified to prescribe narcotics and maintain a license. Other states like Georgia have passed or proposed bills or legislation similar to the Georgia House Bill 400 or The Opioid Abuse and Prevention Act, which requires treatment with non-narcotics before attempting opioids treatment which must be limited for seven days. Also, patients must be educated about the risks of opioids. The prescribers must be able to accept and or properly dispose of unused opioids (the Bill was not passed). Some of these bills and similar bills in different states were defeated, while others were successful. It also appears that some states are creating laws or rules addressing, or adapting the CDC's 2016 guidelines for opioid prescriptions.

The Secure and Responsible Drug Disposal Act of 2010

With respect to the disposal of unused narcotics and other controlled substances, the DEA made available for its implementation The Secure and Responsible Drug Disposal Act of 2010, also called the Disposal Act, which amended the **Controlled Substances Act (CSA) of 1970** giving the DEA the authority to regulate how unused narcotics are disposed of.

The primary objective of this was to control diversions.[5] The CSA was intended to reduce or eliminate diversions by controlling the number of narcotics available and are prescribed.

There are established collection points or sites throughout the country that are registered with the DEA to collect unused controlled substances for destruction.

With the opioid epidemic being of major concern in addition to issues related to the diversions of narcotics, the expectation is that more sites will be registered for collections. The DEA designated two days each year refer to as **National Prescription Drug Take Back Day**. This is discussed in chapter 5.

States Have Enacted Laws that Allow "Harm Reduction Organizations" to Function

Some states have enacted laws that allow "harm reduction organizations" to operate without individuals associated with the organization being subjected to prosecution or becoming part of criminal charges. These are organizations that will provide services such as syringe/needle exchange, education, and others to at-risk groups and individuals. This is intended to reduce the potential spread of infectious diseases (such as hepatitis and HIV), and of course, overdoses and deaths from the opioid epidemic.[14]

Published Guidelines for Opioid Use and Prescription

The CDC and the VA have released guidelines for opioid prescriptions intended mainly for primary care physicians and family medicine physicians/providers who are responsible for more than half of the opioids prescribed in the United States. There are a number of guidelines published by various medical/scientific organizations with similar objectives to the CDC and VA guidelines.[15,31] Also, with respect to treatment, there are several programs and/or other guidelines that were established by the government: these include the aforementioned medication Assisted Treatment (MAT) and Risk Evaluation and Mitigation Strategy (REMS).

Federal Laws Against Designer Drugs

With respect to designer/analog drugs, and considering the overwhelming number of designer drugs and the continuous attempts to make more of them, the federal government passed **The Federal Analog Act, 21 U.S.C § 813** in 1986, making it illegal to manufacture designer/analog compounds that are similar to illegal drugs.

This means that, for example, if someone is trying to manufacture an illegal drug similar in structure, properties or function to a known Schedule I drug, the new drug (although unknown to the federal government/DEA) will also be an illegal Schedule I drug. Therefore, the same laws would apply to the new drug as for the known drugs after which the new one was manufactured to be comparable.[5]

The Stop the Importation of Trafficking of Synthetic Analogs Act (SITSA Act) of 2017

On June 15, 2018, the US House of Representatives voted and passed the SITSA Act of 2017, with 239 for and 142 against. This bill was passed in the Senate. It will strengthen/amend the CSA. In part, one of the objectives of this law is to further empower law enforcement and government agencies in reducing the number of synthetic opioids that are available or may become available. Currently, the largest one, with respect to the opioid epidemic, is the synthetic analogs of IMF, which was responsible for the death of more than 19,000 people in 2016.

The DEA is expected to add a separate class called **Schedule A** to the existing class of drug schedules I-V. This new class will be an illegal class of drugs, including synthetic analogs and any substance deemed necessary or fitting into the category as determined by the DEA and related agencies.[16]

Concerns have been raised by users of **Kratom**; an herb believed to be an "opioid" by some in the government sector and others. The FDA essentially considers kratom and its compounds as opioids. This means that it or its components have the same ability and/or functions that traditional opioids have. Hence, its potential for abuse, use, misuse, and addiction is similar. The DEA has previously released publications indicating that Kratom is similar to opioids in its chemical constituents. In addition to Kratom, other herbs and possibly some supplements that some people believe may be alternative to opioids are now considered at risk to be classified as Schedule A drugs.[17] Of course, there is another side to the story as well, as some believe that this law will help Kratom.[18]

Naloxone Access laws

Making Naloxone More Accessible Regarding treatment: all states have laws that make naloxone/Narcan available and readily accessible for treating users who've had an opioid overdose. This is generally referred to as the **Naloxone Access laws**.

The laws are essentially similar but vary from state to state, with the primary goal being in most instances to make naloxone more easily accessible when treatment needs to be administered.[19,20,21,22]

The Good Samaritan Laws

The Good Samaritan laws, enacted in most states, are designed to decriminalize the victims as well as individuals administering life-saving measures during overdoses. The victims and the persons administering life-saving measures in the presence of illegal drugs may be immune from criminal charges and prosecution. However, each state is different, and it is essential that you know your state's laws and regulations.[23,24,25,26]

H.R. 6, Substance Use-Disorder Prevention that Promotes Opioid Recovery and Treatment (SUPPORT) for Patients and Communities Act

This bill was passed by the House of Representatives on Friday, June 22, 2018, by a vote of 396 to 14. It was introduced on June 13, 2018, by Rep. Greg Walden (R- OR). In part, it will provide more financial support to programs like Medicare and Medicaid as well as to law enforcement agencies in an effort to help combat the opioid epidemic. In particular, law enforcement agencies will be better equipped to deal with the trafficking of drugs such as IMF.

With respect to community involvement or provisions, the mid-levels – physician assistants and nurse practitioners as well as certified nurses – will be able to write prescriptions for substance use disorder.[27]

The Drug Addiction Treatment Act of 2000 (DATA 2000)

Thee DATA 2000 legislation, which is part of the **Children's Health Act of 2000**, was introduced in 2000 by Senators Orrin Hatch, Joe Biden, and Carl Levin. This law permits physicians to treat opioid-addicted or substance use disorder patients.

Physicians must be credentialed and obtain certification for addiction medicine by approval organizations such as the American Board of Medical Specialties or the American Society of

Addiction Medicine. Physicians are allowed to treat these patients with medications approved by the FDA at facilities other than Certified Opioid Treatment Programs.

The DATA 2000 also allows qualified physicians to obtain a waiver that is different from that required by the **Narcotic Addict Treatment Act of 1974**. This permitted the use of treatment with Schedule III-IV and V medications, as was initially done for methadone treatment facilities that require special licensing. DATA 2000 has been amended, and now allows for physicians and mid- levels to treat addicted patients at levels of 30, 100 or 275 patients. Individually, each provider can treat according to their level and experience, with an appropriate waiver even within a group practice. Before the amendment, each group was limited by the number of 30 or 100 patients, regardless of the number of providers in the group.

In 2002, the FDA approved **Suboxone /buprenorphine** to treat substance use disorder at facilities other than Certified Opioid Treatment Programs/Facilities.[28]

Cracking Down on Websites and Stores Illegally Selling Opioids

As the opioid epidemic expands, more and more companies have emerged or are created to capitalize on a market with an expanding base of new consumers or customers. There are many websites and convenience stores that are known to sell controlled substances and/or synthetic analogs of known controlled substances. Sometimes, these are disguised using other names, described as creative labeling or marketing, that may fit into the nutritional supplements or research worlds.

In addition, some of these labels may misrepresent what the initial drug was intended for, which may allow laypersons to diagnose (or misdiagnose) and treat themselves with medications previously expected to be given under the care and supervision or prescribed by physicians/provider only for specific purposes.

The risks are often significant because (among other reasons) sometimes, the individuals consuming these products have no idea of what they are taking, or the appropriate or effective dose in quantities. Sometimes, legally available medication such as opioids and other controlled and noncontrolled substances are available and can be obtained on many websites. The FDA has issued warning letters to more than 50 websites that are either selling or marketing opioids illegally.[30]

The Opioid Crisis Response Act of 2018

The Opioid Crisis Response Act of 2018 Proposals are the result of six bipartisan hearings on the opioid crisis with the FDA, NIH, CDC, SAMHSA, governors, experts, and families. This comprised a package of 70 bills aimed at addressing the opioid epidemic currently impacting our country.[33,34,35]

Thinking outside the Box

A CNBC article reported in part that the FDA had a competition to identify companies that could develop alternative ways to help battle the opioid crisis. FDA is reported to have received more than 250 applications and finally selected eight medical device companies.

Of note is the need or the idea to utilize electronic media, smartphones applications, etc. in hope of helping to control pain. Also, in progress is an effort by the government to work with major social media companies to help in the fight against the opioid epidemic.[13]

References, Recommended Readings and Resources

1. Gery P. Guy Jr., Ph.D.; Kun Zhang, Ph.D.; Michele K. Bohm, MPH; Jan Losby, Ph.D.; Brian Lewis; Randall Young, MA; Louise B. Murphy, Ph.D.; Deborah Dowell, MD. CDCMMWR. Vital Signs: Changes in Opioid Pre- scribing in the United States, 2006–2015. July 7, 2017 / 66(26);697-704. https://www.cdc.gov/mmwr/volumes/66/wr/mm6626a4.htm?s_cid=m- m6626a4_w. Accessed March 1, 2018.

2. Levy B, Paulozzi L, Mack KA, Jones CM. Trends in Opioid Analgesic- Prescribing Rates by Specialty, U.S., 2007-2012. Am J Prev Med. 2015 Sep;49(3):409-13. Apr 18, 2015. Opioid Overdose Prescribing Data. https://www.cdc.gov/drugoverdose/data/prescribing. html. Accessed May 26, 2018.

3. U.S. drug overdose deaths continue to rise; increase fueled by synthetic opioids. https://www.cdc.gov/media/releases/2018/p0329- drug-overdose- deaths.html. Accessed May 5, 2018.

4. Robert W. Patterson. Statement Before the House Judiciary Committee U.S. House of Representatives For a Hearing Entitled: "Challenges and Solutions in the Opioid Abuse Crisis" Presented on May 08, 2018 https:// www.dea.gov/pr/speeches-testimony/2018t/050818t.pdf. Last visited Au- gust 1, 2018.

5. Drug Enforcement Administration. Diversion Control Division. Title 21 United States Code (USC) Controlled Substances Act. Oct. 27, 1986. https://www.deadiversion.usdoj.gov/21cfr/21usc/813.htm. Accessed July 24, 2018.

6. Drug Enforcement Administration: Diversion Control Division. National Prescription Drug Take Back Day.https://www.deadiversion. usdoj.gov/ drug_disposal/takeback/. Last visited July 12, 2018.

7. Pauline Bartolone. Opioid shortages leave US hospitals scrambling. March 19, 2018. https://www.cnn.com/2018/03/19/health/hospital- opioid-short- age-partner/index.html. Accessed on August 1,2018.

8. Comparative Billing Reports. https://www.cbrinfo.net/. Accessed May 31, 2018.

9. 2019 Medicare Advantage and Part D Advance Notice Part II and Draft Call Letter. CMS proposed limits on opioids. https://www.cms.gov/Newsroom/ MediaReleaseDatabase/Fact-sheets/2018-Fact-sheets- items/2018-02-01. html. Accessed July 31,2018.

10. Centers for Disease Control and Prevention. Calculating Morphine Milli- gram Equivalents. https://www.cdc.gov/drugoverdose/pdf/ calculating_total_daily_dose-a.pdf. Accessed May 30,2018.

11. Deborah Dowell, MD; Tamara M. Haegerich, Ph.D.; Roger Chou, MD. CDC Guideline for Prescribing Opioids for Chronic Pain. Morbidity and Mortality Weekly Report (MMWR). March 18,2016. https://www.cdc.gov/ mmwr/volumes/65/rr/rr6501e1.htm. Accessed July 23,2018.

12. Drug Enforcement Administration. Drug Facts Sheet-Narcotics. https:// www.dea.gov/druginfo/drug_data_sheets/Narcotics.pdf. Accessed July 4, 2018.

13. FDA picks eight medical device firms to help battle opioid crisis November 30, 2018. https://www.cnbc.com/2018/11/30/fda-picks-eight- medical-de- vice-firms-to-help-battle-opioid-crisis.html. Accessed December 1,2018.

14. Harm Reduction Coalition. http://harmreduction.org/about-us/ principles-of-harm-reduction/. Accessed July 31, 2018.

15. Deborah Dowell, MD; Tamara M. Haegerich, Ph.D.; Roger Chou, MD. CDC Guideline for Prescribing Opioids for Chronic Pain. Morbidity and Mortality Weekly Report (MMWR). March 18,2016. https://www.cdc.gov/ mmwr/volumes/65/rr/rr6501e1.htm. Accessed July 23,2018.

16. H.R. 2851 – Stop the Importation of Trafficking of Synthetic Analogs Act (SITSA Act). Sponsored by Rep. John Katko (R-NY). https://www.con- gress.gov/bill/115th-congress/house-bill/2851/ text?format=txt. Accessed on June 19,2018.

17. Peter Hess. The House Just Passed a Bill That Could Make Kratom Illegal June 18, 2018. https://www.inverse.com/article/46088-what-is- the-sitsa- act-and-what-does-it-mean-for- kratom. Accessed June 19,2018.

18. National Kratom Coalition supports S.1327/ H. R. 2851. https:// nation-alkratomcoalition.org/the-national-kratom-coalition-supports-s-1327-h-r- 2851-sitsa-act/. Accessed June 19, 2018.

19. Preventing the Consequences of Opioid Overdose: Understanding Naloxone Access Laws.https://www.samhsa.gov/capt/sites/default/ files/resources/naloxone-access-laws- tool.pdf. Accessed March 16, 2018.

20. Susan P Weinstein. Naloxone Access and Good Samaritan Overdose Protection Laws Abound in State Legislatures. June 24, 2015.https:// drugfree. org/learn/drug-and-alcohol-news/commentary-naloxone- access-good-samaritan-overdose-protection-laws-abound-state- legislatures/. Accessed March 16, 2018.

21. Jerome M. Adams, MD, MPH, VADM. Increasing Naloxone Awareness and Use: The Role of Health Care Practitioners. JAMA. 2018;319(20):2073- 2074. May 22/29, 2018. https://jamanetwork.com/ journals/jama/article-abstract/2678206. Accessed on June 30, 2018.

22. Francie Diep. How easy is it to get naloxone in your states? Here's how states have made it easier for bystanders to administer naloxone to overdose victims. April 6, 2018. https://psmag.com/news/how-easy- is-it- to-get-naloxone-in-your-state. Accessed on June 30, 2018.

23. Susan P Weinstein Commentary: Naloxone Access and Good Samaritan Overdose Protection Laws Abound in State Legislatures. June 24, 2015. https://drugfree.org/learn/drug-and-alcohol-news/ commentary-naloxone-access-good-samaritan-overdose-protection- laws-abound-state-legislatures/. Accessed March 16, 2018.

24. Jerome M. Adams, MD, MPH, VADM. Increasing Naloxone Awareness and Use: The Role of Health Care Practitioners. JAMA. 2018;319(20):2073- 2074. May 22/29, 2018. https://jamanetwork.com/ journals/jama/article-abstract/2678206. Accessed on June 30, 2018.

25. The Network for Public Health Law. Legal Interventions to Reduce Over- dose Mortality: Naloxone Access and Overdose Good Samaritan Law. https://www.networkforphl.org/_asset/qz5pvn/legal- interventions-to-reduce-overdose.pdf. Accessed March 16, 2018.

26. Menu of State Laws Related to Prescription Drug Overdose Emergencies. https://www.cdc.gov/phlp/docs/menu-pdoe.pdf. Accessed March 30, 2018.

27. H.R. 6, SUBSTANCE USE-DISORDER PREVENTION THAT PRO- MOTES OPIOID RECOVERY AND TREATMENT (SUPPORT) FOR PATIENTS AND COMMUNITIES ACT. https://policy.house. gov/legislative/bills/hr-6-substance-use-disorder-prevention-promotes-opioid-recovery-and-treatment. Accessed June 23, 2018.

28. Substance Abuse and Mental Health Services Administration. Legislation, Regulations, and Guidelines. https://www.samhsa.gov/ programs-campaigns/medication-assisted-treatment/legislation-regulations-guidelines. Accessed July 3, 2018.

29. Narcotic Addicts Treatment Act of 1974. https://www.gpo.gov/fdsys/ pkg/ STATUTE-88/pdf/STATUTE-88-Pg124.pdf. Accessed July 3, 2018.

30. Opioid-Selling Websites Warned. Practical Pain Management. July 6, 2018. https://www.practicalpainmanagement.com/resources/news-and- research/ opioid-selling-websites-warned. Accessed July 7, 2018.

31. VA/DoD Clinical Practice Guideline for Opioid Therapy For Chronic Pain. December 2016. https://www.healthquality.va.gov/guidelines/Pain/cot/ VADoDOTCPG022717.pdf. Accessed August 1, 2018.

32. Proposed Aggregate Production Quotas for Schedule I and II Controlled Substances and Assessment of Annual Needs for the List I Chemicals Ephedrine, Pseudoephedrine, and Phenylpropanolamine for 2019. August 20, 2018. https://www.deadiversion.usdoj.gov/fed_regs/quotas/2018/ fr0820.htm. Last visited August 21, 2018.

33. The Opioid Crisis Response Act of 2018. https://www.help.senate.gov/ imo/media/doc/The%20Opioid%20Crisis%20Response%20Act%20 of%20 2018%20summary.pdf. Accessed September 23rd, 2018.

34. Colby Itkowitz. Senate passes sweeping opioids package. September 17, 2018. https://www.washingtonpost.com/politics/2018/09/17/senate-set-pass-sweeping-opioids-package/?noredirect=on&utm_term=.6ee- bc41a1f68. Accessed September 23, 2018.

35. Michael Collins. USA Today. Senate advances plan to combat opioid epidemic. Sept. 17, 2018. https://www.usatoday.com/story/news/ pol- itics/2018/09/17/opioid-crisis-senate-bill-stems-flow-drugs-offers-treatment-access/1270720002/. Accessed September 23, 2018.

Chapter 17

Trust but Verify: When Your Doctor Cannot Help You or You Have No Doctor

"Trust but Verify" – Pres. Ronald Reagan

Something to believe in is good, someone to believe in is truly awesome. When it comes to life and death, it is so important to know that the information you have is correct and that you can count on as well as depend on the source of that information. We should always feel entrusted to look out and care for the ones we love or hold close to our hearts. Whether it be your children or your loved ones, when it gets to that point in their life when the truth is only an option and not their defining principle, you have an obligation to ensure that the information you get from them can be relied on or is accurate. In other words, you must verify.

The mindset of an addict or a substance use disorder individual isn't that of the person who existed before it. Individuals who are caught up in the web of substance use disorder, often by compulsion, desire and the need to survive, find it absolutely necessary to do what they think is in their best interest. This usually means getting drugs. Therefore, it doesn't matter what your perspective or position is, or what your rights and beliefs are; all of that becomes secondary to them. Therefore, manipulation, lies, and deceit are expected; and is generally the norm.

One of the adverse effects of opioids on individuals who are addicts or opioid dependents is a decline in the cognitive function of the brain; the frontal-lobe deficit primarily increases. This affects the brain and the individual's ability to process and function in ways that are typically considered rational and objective. It is not uncommon for addicts to lose their sense of reality and become reckless, with no regard to the consequence of their actions.[1,2,3,4]

As you look out for one another and the people you care about, simply ask yourself, "do you trust the drug dealers or drug suppliers?"

The overwhelming objective of drug dealers and suppliers is to make money. They could care less about whether or not users live or die; as long as they make money, they will have accomplished their goals.

Dealers and suppliers will always add additives or fillers to drugs to make them stronger and, more importantly, to increase the quantity of drugs available for sale. Therefore, a drug dealer will always find something to add to, for example, legal powdered substances or illegal fentanyl or heroin to increase both volume and profit margin. Sometimes, the purchasers of the drugs may get something that could or do kill them. They may get something that is of poor quality or does not represent what it is supposed to be. So, the buyers of drugs will always be at a disadvantage that can typically and often leads to death from overdose. This may also lead to medical complications and other issues related to ingesting substances in their body that were not intended for human consumption. If someone you know is purchasing drugs from dealers and suppliers or wherever, simply ask them: "how can they trust someone who could do anything with the drugs they are buying, therefore putting their lives at risk?" The next big question is, of course: "how do you verify anything?"

To opioid addicts, it will make very little difference or none at all. Their primary goal is to fulfill their craving for a specific substance. They'll do whatever it takes or accept whatever is offered to them to satisfy their needs.

A similar but different example of this is the so-called **pharming party**; here, individuals will bring prescription medications as well as over-the-counter medications such as cough/cold medicines to a party, and put them all in one container from which those present at the party can take from it and ingest. Of course, the significant danger here is that these people often do not know what they're ingesting, and neither do they know the risks or danger involved.

In addition to ingesting unknown medications, other substances such as alcohol or other illegal drugs may be involved, thereby compounding the problem. If opioids are present (and they often are), this can also lead to a potential overdose that may lead to death, which is exactly what has happened on numerous occasions.

The Discharge Process

The patient-doctor relationship is indeed very special. The doctor has a responsibility (at the very least) to provide the utmost care for each of his or her patients to be well while maintaining confidentiality without regard to financial ability, race, class, sexual orientation, religion, etc.

The patients have the responsibility to be honest, truthful, and provide the best possible information to their doctors or healthcare providers to facilitate the best possible care.

In the world of pain management best practice, the relationship begins with a contractual agreement between the provider and patients, referred to as the **pain management agreement**. Each patient is expected to abide by this agreement or be subjected to possible discharge from the care of their providers if an amicable resolution cannot be obtained after a breach was identified.

The agreement spells out how and under what terms opioids or other controlled substances will be prescribed, and the requirements that are necessary for the physician to continue treating the patients. I have enclosed what is considered a standard discharge/separation letter and the end of this chapter.

One of the most challenging processes for most pain management specialists is finding common ground where you can realistically treat, monitor and provide the best possible care to your patients. Thus, without putting yourself or your practice at risk because of patients' unacceptable and risky behavior, or enabling or facilitating patient-care that will ultimately result in patients' self-destructing conduct.

Patients who present to pain management practices with a very high dose (an MME greater than 100 or more) of opioids and are chronic users most often believe that because they have been using or have been prescribed a high dose of opioids, they are entitled to continue on the same dose.

They're usually very resistant to change and are frequently discharged for noncompliance because of overtaking or failing to follow what is expected of them. They tend to fall into **Class III** and **IV** of **FOCAS**.

Some discharged patients test positive for illegal drugs such as cocaine, methamphetamine, heroin, and others. However, they deny knowing how it got into their system. They are not usually willing to participate in a drug recovery program. They, therefore, continue to seek other providers in the hope of finding their desired combination or amount of opioids. However, failing to do that result in them going deeper into crisis by using illicit drugs like heroin, illegally manufactured drugs like fentanyl or designer drugs. When no doctor fulfills their needs, they often find a drug dealer or someone who will temporarily facilitate their drug need or dependence, or substance use disorder/addiction.

Some patients will attempt to get prescriptions from multiple doctors or from individuals who have obtained prescriptions from opioid diversions.

Their UDTs are often negative or tampered with. They are unwilling to participate in any other program that will result in the reduction of opioids. These programs may include physical therapy, cognitive behavioral therapy, and psychotherapy. They tend to refuse even diagnostic tests, or any intervention or therapeutic modality that will alleviate pain. They will refuse joint injections and spinal injections that are warranted and proven to be beneficial in helping reduce pain and opioid use. To top it off, only specific opioids work for them in specific doses; and other medications (called adjuvants) will have some serious side effects, except for their benzos and alcohol.

Another category of patients is made up of those who appear to be compliant and participating in occasional treatments/programs. They have figured out all the relevant tools used in pain management and how to beat the system. They'll have normal or consistent UDTs as well as confirmation studies, they'll do well on their pill counts, and their SPDMP data will be okay.

However, an experienced pain management provider, considering all the factors associated with this group of patients, may decide to discharge them from the practice because, in their judgment, they pose risks both to themselves and the practice. Patients have the right to discharge or change physicians/providers, and physicians/providers have the right to discharge patients whom they do not feel comfortable treating them. This may lead to discharge from the physician with a simple reason:

"Dr. John no longer feels comfortable providing care for you."

Another important factor for those trying so hard to be helpful in their loved ones' or significant others' lives, is paying attention to patients' **reason for discharge**. Now, of course, you cannot call the patient's doctor and try to elicit information about the patient because that will not be given to you due to confidentiality. However, be aware that almost all good pain management practices have very good reasons to discharge patients. There are times when, and this happens most of the time, these are early signs of trouble for the discharged individuals.

These events may be the result of the patients' abusing prescription drugs and/or opioids; they may have illicit drugs such as cocaine, marijuana, methamphetamine or others in their system. They might have been obtaining multiple prescriptions of opioids and/or other medications from several doctors/providers. They are probably excessively overusing or abusing prescribed medications from their pain management doctors/providers.

Sometimes they may be discharged after failed repeated attempts for them to follow through on recommended treatments such as seeing psychologists, psychiatrists, and other consultants; or obtaining appropriate tests.

Always remember that pain management is not just about giving opioids; it is essential that patients follow through on the recommendations that are made in order for them to obtain effective treatment while being treated in pain management practice. This is necessary for them to be on the path of recovery and to significantly reduce the risk of developing opioid dependence or opioid use disorder.

The discharge of patients from management practices often provide an opportunity to begin a dialogue, with the goal of establishing clear reasons for discharge. Sometimes, discharges are the first sign that some form of intervention may be necessary, which at this stage will be much easier and more effective. What's important here is for you to have clear and verifiable information as to why your significant others, loved ones or those you care about were discharged. It is not good enough to just accept their word, because at this point their word may be meaningless, particularly if they are opioid-dependent or addicted.

They are more likely to lie, manipulate, or deceive. Therefore, the time of discharge should provide the opportunity to discuss with your loved ones and significant others what is really happening.

Almost everyone who has been discharged from a pain management clinic is given a discharge letter or statement; this often explains why the patient was discharged. This, however, will also have information that will vary in content and detail, depending on the pain management clinics. This will be a starting point to ascertain meaningful information to provide a better understanding of what is happening in the lives of your significant others. If you have a good relationship with your loved ones or significant others, children and others you may be responsible for, this moment could provide the best time to talk about these issues and seek additional help. However, never be happy or satisfied with simple answers such as: "they" don't know what they're doing, their staff are rude, they only want my money, they are not helping me with my pain, there is a better doctor or facility on the other side of town (which may be miles away from where they usually have to travel).

Always remember that almost everyone who is discharged has been discharged for a very good reason.

How About Kicking Grandma
Out or Throwing Grandpa Out of the Practice?

Okay, that is probably too mean, or someone may see this as encouraging elderly abuse. So, we'll just settle for discharging grandma and grandpa from the practice. Before I was involved in pain management, I worked in geriatric facilities and rehabilitation centers. Generally, it would have been hard to understand why patients in their 70s, 80s, and 90s indirectly or directly contribute to the opioid epidemic. The reality is that there are so many individuals (ranging from children, grandchildren or their relatives and caregivers) who continuously abuse and use the elderly to obtain narcotics and controlled substances. It is reasonable to believe that as one gets older, it is likely that they will have a greater need for pain control. As such, many older patients are prescribed a significant number of opioids and controlled substances, only for the drugs to be taken away from them by the perpetrators for their own personal use or desires.

These older patients then show up at the clinic with inconsistent urine, pill counts, multiple prescribers, and the presence in their system of illegal drugs ranging from cocaine, marijuana, methamphetamines and more.

Moreover, when these things are discovered, and it is clear that there is abuse, although we are limited by what we can say or divulge to protective services, we can still alert them for what is often described as the **"Well-Care Check"** in the hope that these older (and often, entirely dependent) patients will be cared for appropriately. Hence, because of the gravity of the situation and similar issues, these patients have to be discharged from the practice. Aside from the abuse that often takes place, there are some willing and able participants who often work in conjunction with their relatives or caregiver to get opioids/controlled substances that they are not taking, but are subsequently diverged. As we strive to protect and treat the elderly in our care for the pain they do have, we must also remember that old age does not necessarily correlate with innocence.

Also, we must not forget that the elderly and cognitively impaired patients with psychiatric disorders and physically/functionally challenged patients, among others, are frequently used and abused to obtain opioids and other controlled substances for caregivers or relatives.

One of the most unfortunate things in the discharge process is not being able to take care of the ones who need it most. Often, it is simply because they are in denial, they don't care, they're ashamed and defiant.

They are at a place in their lives where they do not see themselves as having a problem, and therefore in their minds, they do not need treatment or help from anyone.

Whether their physicians or providers discharge them or they simply do not return to the practice, it is truly very sad. Another sad process in the discharge process is discharging patients who simply failed to be truthful or honest in explaining inconsistencies in their history regarding how they take their medications or having urine drug tests that are inconsistent with their history. My best advice to them is simple; be truthful and honest with your doctors or medical providers. If we have to become detectives and make great efforts to figure out how or why there is inconsistency in their history then it is so much easier and appropriate to discharge patients that fit this scenario. We can be of much greater help to them if we know the truth, believe it or not, pain management providers truly want to be at their service, but they have to play their part.

On the next page is an example of a discharge letter or separation notice. Patients are generally given one of these, or one is mailed to them. As indicated above, the format and content vary widely.

References, Recommended Readings and Resources

1. Thomas Kosten, Tony P George. The Neurobiology of Opioid Dependence: Implications for Treatment. NIH. Science & Practice Perspectives. 13-20. August 2002. https://www.researchgate.net/ publication/5288549_The_ Neurobiology_of_Opioid_Dependence_ Implications_for_Treatment. Accessed July 7, 2018.
2. National Institute on Drug Abuse. Principles of Drug Addiction Treatment: A Research-Based Guide. Third edition. Last reviewed December 2012. https://www.drugabuse.gov/sites/default/files/ podat_1.pdf. Accessed July 2, 2018.
3. George F. Koob. The neurobiology of addiction: a neuroadaptational view relevant for diagnosis. 08 August 2006. https://onlinelibrary. wiley.com/ doi/abs/10.1111/j.1360-0443.2006.01586.x. Accessed June 30, 2018.
4. George F Koob Ph.D., Nora D Volkow MD. Neurobiology of addiction: a neurocircuitry analysis. The Lancet Psychiatry. Volume 3, Issue 8, August 2016, Pg. 760-773. https://www.sciencedirect.com/ science/article/pii/ S2215036616001048. Accessed on June 30, 2018.

EXAMPLE   **PRACTICE'S INFORMATION**
DISCHARGE/SEPARATION LETTER

Patient's Name: Joe Goodbye   DOB:_____DATE: _____

This letter is to inform you that we will no longer provide Pain Management/ Medical Services for you. The condition(s) upon which you have been discharged is described below:

- Failure to maintain scheduled appointments.

- Failure to comply with the recommended treatment plan to reduce your use of narcotics.

- Receiving multiple prescriptions from multiple providers.

- Refused to cooperate with Patient Billing Services Department.

- Dr. Provider is no longer comfortable providing pain management services to you.

- Patient requests voluntary dismissal from Center for Pain and Rehab Medicine.

- Your prescribed medications were not present in your drug screen.

- You had an additional non-disclosed medication present in your drug screen that was not prescribed by Dr. Provider.

- Illegal substance (cocaine) was found in your drug screen. You should report to a drug treatment facility immediately for rehabilitation.

- Improper use, abuse or dependence of prescribed medication(s).

- Other.

It is recommended that you promptly find another doctor/intervention as all future appointments have been cancelled. I will make myself available to you for 30 days on an emergency basis only. During this time, I will be unable to prescribe you any pain medications. If you have an emergency while waiting for an appointment with another facility, you should go to the nearest emergency room for treatment.

Respectfully,
Dr. Treating Provider

INTERVENTION	PHONE NUMBER	WEB ADDRESS
Alcoholic Anonymous	404-525-3178	www.atlantaaaa.org
Domestic Violence	800-334-2836	www.pady.org
Narcotic Anonymous	404-708-3215	www.na.org
Suicide Hotline	800-784-2433	www.suicidehotlines.com

Part Four

MOVING FORWARD, BECAUSE THAT IS WHAT WE DO. WE WILL, AND WE MUST PREVAIL.

Chapter 18

Are We Providing Doctors and Medical and Service Providers with All the Tools and Support Required to Make Them Effective in the Opioid Epidemic?

The opioid epidemic is one of the single most significant crises this country has faced in many generations. Of course, efforts are being made at every degree to combat and bring this crisis to a halt. Admittedly, there have been strides made in helping to provide additional services and funding to facilitate healthcare providers and service-related providers with essential tools to fight this epidemic. But is this enough? Moreover, how are the personnel involved in coping with and addressing the needs required to make a difference in dealing with this epidemic?

Here are some of the concerns and issues of most medical providers and healthcare service personnel which limits or, in some ways, restricts our effectiveness in better caring for and managing the challenges involved in taking care of opioid patients and potential users.

Consider the following:

A 36-year-old female had surgery to remove her ovaries and uterus. However, she developed abdominal pain and was started and maintained on Percocet 10/325 mg four times a day around-the-clock for six months. She presented to a clinic with a referral for pain management, with a diagnosis of opioid dependence. The decision was made in part to decrease her Percocet to 7.5/325 mg at three times a day, and add a **Butrans Patch** (10 µg) once weekly along with other supporting or adjuvant medications such as muscle relaxer, anti-inflammatory, and neuropathic medications.

The intention was to gradually wean her off or reduce the amount of opioids she was taking. **The healthcare insurance company** responded by saying it does not cover **Butrans Patch**. However, **fentanyl or Morphine, which are part of their formulary medications, will be covered and is recommended**.

Now, this case is not unique in of itself. However, if the best option is always the cheapest option, without consideration of the effects that the medications will have on patients, the opioid epidemic will likely have more patients available to increase its numbers. I'm not taking the position that I agree or disagree with the treatment. But the significant issue here is that we are talking about improving the opioid epidemic and finding ways to decrease the use of certain types of opioids, primarily Schedule II extended-release or long-acting drugs that are generally more addictive. Probably because of the economic costs, the healthcare insurance company was not willing to cover the medication that is more effective, more beneficial and probably less likely to worsen the opioid epidemic, leading to a better outcome than the one that was recommended.

A 40-year-old male was being followed by a pain management clinic and was taking hydrocodone 10/325 mg four to six times a day. Healthcare providers/ physicians have some concern that there may be a risk for diversion. He wanted to prescribe an **opioid abuse-deterrent formulation (Hysingla ER, Embeda, Morphabond ER, or Xtampza ER)**, and none of them was approved by the patient's healthcare insurance. Again, a recommendation was made for Fentanyl Patch or Morphine Sulfate ER as choices for long-acting/extended- release opioid medication.

This case, and so many like it, comes down to money, and who is willing to pay or who is responsible. The abuse-deterrent formulations would fill the need for reducing the risks of diversions and the number of pills available for the patients' use. At the same time, they can provide more than adequate treatment for pain. Of course, they do not eliminate the risks of diversions or misuse and abuse of opioids, but several studies show that these medications are effective in reducing or helping to reverse the opioid epidemic by decreasing the overall risks.

The irony of this whole process is that opioids like fentanyl, oxycodone, and morphine, which are most significantly associated with exacerbating the opioid epidemic, are the ones on formulary lists and are recommended by a significant number of healthcare insurance companies. Although fentanyl is generally prescribed as a transdermal patch to the public, it is extremely dangerous if it is used inappropriately or misused.

The fentanyl that is most commonly associated with opioid overdose and deaths is IMF, usually in the form of powder or pills that can be made into a solution. Fentanyl, in general, is about 50 times as potent as heroin and is extremely deadly as its users have created different mixtures along with other substances/ drugs (both legal and illegal) which are then ingested.

In some states, there are healthcare insurance companies whose formulary medications include methadone as a long-acting/extended-release instead of the abuse-deterrent formulations. This, in essence, has the potential to create a class of methadone-addicted patients who were never on heroin. Some of these patients do eventually end up in methadone clinics for treatment of their chronic pain. **Butrans patch** (buprenorphine) is considered another abuse-deterrent formulation which is applied to the skin (transdermal) once weekly. It is frequently denied by a large number of insurance companies.[1]

Ms. Thomas, a 60+-year-old female, has been managed by a pain management clinic. She has had chronic pain for more than eight years and is on high-dose opioids. She had an X-ray of her back, which shows arthritis. Her **healthcare insurance company will not approve physical therapy because her condition is chronic**. The healthcare insurance company will also not approve an MRI of her lower back unless she has physical therapy. So, what are the options of the health care provider?

Should he or she continue opioids without any reasonable way of managing the patient, or is it fair to discharge this patient because as the healthcare provider, you are unable to effectively or appropriately treat this patient without continuing to give opioids with a high probability of dose escalations?

Issues like these may not seem like major problems. However, they can be extremely frustrating to both patients and healthcare providers. Of course, not every patient who has chronic pain will necessarily need an MRI or a CT scan for their treatment to be effective. Also, sometimes there may be some other diagnostic tests that may be useful, even if to a lesser degree. However, understanding what's being treated and the probable reasons for the patient's pain will ultimately result in better care and utilization of services for patients' management.

The Need for Mental Disorder Care

The need for mental disorder care has always been a significant one in this country. Very often, individuals with mental illness/behavioral health issues are not treated appropriately or adequately for a plethora of reasons.

This may include finances or the lack thereof, the stigma attached to mental/behavioral illness, limited resources available to behavioral/mental healthcare providers, and a significant shortage of providers.

In the field of pain management, there is and always will be a growing need for the services of healthcare providers for mental/behavioral illness. So often, it is difficult to find providers who could deal with the ever-increasing number of patients who need care while under the care of pain management.[3,4,5]

It has been reported that more than 51% of the prescribed opioids in the United States are prescribed to patients with mental illness disorders.[6] However, there never seems to be enough providers who can provide the required service. Also, the amount of funds allocated for treating mental/behavioral illness is usually considered small relative to the existing need. Some healthcare insurance companies have very little coverage for mental/behavioral illness treatments such as psychotherapy/behavioral therapy. In addition, the reimbursement rates paid to behavioral/mental health providers are often considered among the lowest in the healthcare sector.[4,5]

The Denial of Interventional Procedures

The denial of interventional procedures for pain management is often a frequent complaint of many pain management providers. It is not uncommon for procedures such as epidural injections, nerve blocks, joint injections, spinal cord stimulator implants, and many others to be denied.

The denial of service by healthcare insurance occurs for so many different reasons, poor or inadequate documentation is very common is one of them. Sometimes, they frequently use terms like 'experimental' and/or 'investigative,' with not enough evidence to support the procedure. However, even when documentation and medical conditions are appropriate, there is still a significant number of denials for important procedures. These procedures have been shown over the years through scientific research data and clinical outcomes to be very effective. They often have been shown to reduce pain significantly, and hence, also decrease the need for opioids or controlled substances.

These treatment options can in some instances result in patients being opioid-free. Sometimes, the reasons for the denial are justified, but what is seen very often by a significant number of pain management practices and other specialties are what appear to be random or arbitrary denials for no apparent or valid reason. This is sometimes resolved by what is called a peer-to-peer review that may require about 15 minutes to half an hour to be usually completed by telephone. Although this may not seem like a significant amount of time, the complaint form most practices are that it is a considerable (but probably necessary) burden; and often results in delays of service or services not rendered because of the initial denials.

Patients sometimes are most helpful in that they can call their healthcare insurance companies, which helps facilitate the process.

In general, wherever appropriate and, relevant services that can be provided to reduce the dependence on opioids should be strongly encouraged and facilitated, as we all struggle to take control of the opioid epidemic and the major healthcare crisis that has resulted because of it.

There are Many Topical Medications

Many topical medications are often very effective and useful for treating pain. However, these are usually not covered by most insurance companies as they are considered too expensive. Most of them are non-narcotic, non-addictive and often very safe, without any major systemic effect. This can be particularly useful in the elderly population, where patients usually do not tolerate systemic medications very well.

In addition, most elderly patients are usually on so many other medications that they are taking orally. Therefore, adding a patch is often very helpful. Topical medications including pain cream, compounded medications, ointment, and non- opioid pain patches have been found to be very useful.

These scenarios do not apply to all healthcare insurance companies but do apply to a significant number that potentially has a negative impact on how patients are managed, as well as affect the long-term probability of increasing the number of patients subsequently considered or diagnosed as substance use disorder patients. Although healthcare insurance is a business, the goal of healthcare providers and insurance companies must consider the long-term effect that some decisions have not only on providers' ability to manage patients but on the overall outcome of patients' medical conditions.

Therefore, if medical providers and other healthcare providers are required to uphold a certain standard and be responsible or accountable for the opioid epidemic and all the challenges that it brings, then all healthcare insurance companies who are collecting premiums and not paying their fair share should also have a responsibility to do so.

The Denial of UDT

The task of reversing the opioid epidemic requires many different and effective tools and options. We had talked in this book about the SPDMP, medication reviews, following appropriate guidelines for opioid prescriptions, and the proper evaluation and treatment of patients with alternatives other than opioids wherever possible, among other things.[7]

The use of **UDT** still remains one of the most objective tools available to identify patients who are misusing or abusing opioids/other controlled substances, as well as monitoring them therapeutically.

Most pain management practices strive to find the most effective way of utilizing this method to its best productive effect. There are currently no official guidelines established by any specific entity that clearly defines how and when these tests should be done and the most appropriate reasons for doing so.

The CMS has established guidelines related to the various coverage areas of the country. However, most insurance companies have established their own guidelines, which do not fully take into account the needs of the patients or the scientific bases of testing, particularly when it pertains to definitive testing or confirmation testing.[10]

Their guidelines and regulations or protocols appear to be based primarily on the financial priorities or needs of the health insurance companies. They will change their policies and regulations regarding UDT at any time by limiting appropriate testing to a minimum for even patients who are very complex or considered high-risk. This often leads to chaos because there are no standard protocols or guidelines that healthcare providers/physicians, healthcare insurance companies, and governmental insurance are required to follow. This results in frequent denials of UDT that are appropriate for the patients being tested.

Of course, there are abuses in the system by some healthcare providers/ physicians and major laboratory companies and reference labs. These abuses often make it difficult for the legitimate testing of deserving patients and negatively impact the management of patients who are taking opioids. Therefore, they are abused by the providers/physicians on one side, and by the healthcare insurance companies and the providers/physicians on the other side.

They simply do this by making and manipulating their own rules and regulation, and in so doing, deny legitimate claims. This makes it harder for patients to be monitored and managed appropriately while being treated with opioid medications as well as other controlled substances. Hence, the opioid epidemic can be made worse by the actions of some healthcare insurance companies who fail to appropriately cover the costs of UDT necessary to monitor each patient and ensure that they are compliant while on opioid medications.

Clearly, the opioid epidemic can be reversed at least in part with more significant support and major contributions for coverage of the cost of alternative medicine and pain treatment such as behavioral therapy, physical therapy, spinal intervention procedures, and appropriate mental disorder treatment instead of major doses of opioids. In addition, diagnostic testing such as X-ray, CT scan, MRI and EMG/nerve conduction studies, and laboratory testing are but some of the things that play an integral and positive part in significantly affecting this opioid epidemic.

Monitoring Frequency and Frequency

The terms monitoring frequency, medical necessity, and frequency are often used in the care and treatment of most patients. These terms are often considered self- explanatory. However, when used in the treatment and management of patients, there are often blurred lines. This occurs between what is medically necessary, or how frequently particular procedures or tests should be done, and the type of monitoring appropriate for the specialty or the condition being treated.

In addition, the patient population being treated comes into play. Of course, the patient's condition being treated and the supporting documents often determine or clarify the need or justification for any of these terms.[10]

The CDC's 2016 (intended for primary care providers) indicated that monitoring frequency in the form of a re-evaluation and face-to-face appointments by the prescriber is recommended every 90 days for patients receiving greater than 50 MMEs, and every 30 days for patients receiving greater than 120 MME.[11] This is definitely an improvement from what typically happens, where patients receiving opioids are given multiple refills for an extended period without being evaluated and examined until their next 90, 180 or more days have elapsed before they are seen for follow-up treatment.

There are many questions, some of which are: what happens during the 90- or 30-day period when these patients are in the so-called free world? Are they still compliant?

How frequently are they urine-tested? Are they given any other options than opioids? But probably the most significant question is: how trustworthy are these patients who are on opioids?

In general, it can be said that probably most patients will do the right thing and follow instructions, and take their medication as prescribed, without diversions or misuse and abuse. However, the experience most of us in pain management has is different. We see a significant number of pain management patients and even more non-pain management patients that if they are not properly supervised or monitored, they are most likely the ones who will be most dishonest. They will use every opportunity to abuse the system and some providers' naiveté by simply doing whatever they can get away with. It is clearly not enough to see these patients face-to-face and evaluate them without random UDT, medications review, planned reduction of opioid use, or implementing other means of reducing pain other than opioids. [11]

The hard and unfortunate reality is that monitoring patients frequently and ensuring that they are compliant with their use of opioids is an expensive process, which no one at this time is willing to pay for.

It appears that the cost of treatment that is meaningful and helpful in the reduction of the opioid epidemic is beyond most healthcare insurance company budgets as well as governmental insurances that have always had funding challenges.

An NIH article stated that the CDC has estimated that the total economic burden of prescription opioid misuse alone in the United States is $78.5 billion a year, including the cost of healthcare, lost productivity, addiction treatment, and criminal justice involvement. However, The Council of Economic Advisers or National Economic Council stated in November 2017 that the cost in 2015 for the opioid epidemic or crisis was $504 billion. [9] In that year alone, 33,000 people died from an opioid overdose. So where will the extra funding required to fight this epidemic come from? In 2016, about 42,000 individuals died from an opioid- related overdose. [8] Clearly, the costs of this epidemic are expected to rise every year, along with the death toll. Regardless of what the figures are and once they are straightened out, it will be an ever-increasing significant cost to our economy. Who will pay and where will they get the funds from?

References, Recommended Readings and Resources

1. Katie Thomas and Charles Ornstein September 17, 2017. Amid Opioid Crisis, Insurers Restrict Pricey, Less Addictive Painkillers. https:// www. nytimes.com/2017/09/17/health/opioid-painkillers-insurance- companies. html. Accessed March 7, 2018

2. Stacy Weiner, Association of American Colleges News. Addressing the Escalating Psychiatrist Shortage. February 13, 2018. https://news. aamc.org/patient-care/article/addressing-escalating-psychiatrist- shortage/. Accessed June 16, 2018.

3. Bruce Japsen, Forbes. Psychiatrist Shortage Escalates as U.S. Mental Health Needs Grow. Feb 25, 2018. https://www.forbes. com/forbes/welcome/?toURL=https://www.forbes.com/sites/brucejapsen/2018/02/25/psychiatrist-shortage-escalates-as-u-s-mental-health-needs-grow/&re-fURL=https://www.google. com/&referrer=https://www.google.com/. Accessed May 5, 2018.

4. Lizzie O'Leary and Peter Balonon-Rosen, Marketplace. When it comes to insurance money, mental health is not treated equal. January 05, 2018. https://www.marketplace.org/2018/01/05/health-care/ doctors-get-more- insurance-money-psychiatrists-when-treating- mental-health. Accessed June 16, 2018

5. Alana Carvalho, HuffPost. Stop Insurance Companies from Discriminating Against Mental Health Patients. 08/18/2017. https:// www.huffington- post.com/entry/stop-insurance-companies-from- discriminating-against_ us_59971709e4b03b5e472cef04. Accessed June 16, 2018.

6. Matthew A. Davis, MPH, Ph.D., Lewei A. Lin, MD, Haiyin Liu, MA, and Brian D. Sites, MD, MS. Prescription Opioid Use among Adults with Mental Health Disorders in the United States. June 26, 2017. https://kai- serhealthnews.files.wordpress.com/2017/06/opioidembargo- article.pdf. Accessed August 2, 2018.

7. Matthew J. Bair MD, MS, Erin E. Krebs MD, MPH. Pain Practice: Why Is Urine Drug Testing Not Used More Often in Practice? November/December 2010. Pages 493-496. https://onlinelibrary.wiley. com/doi/full/10.1111/ j.1533-2500.2010.00425.x. Accessed March 20, 2018.

8. NIH, Opioid overdose crisis.https://www.drugabuse.gov/drugs-abuse/ opioids/opioid-overdose-crisis. Accessed June 4, 2018.

9. The Underestimated Cost of the Opioid Crisis. The Economic Advisory Council November 2017. https://www.whitehouse.gov/sites/ whitehouse. gov/files/images/The%20Underestimated%20Cost%20 of%20the%20Opi-oid%20Crisis.pdf. Accessed June 15, 2018.

10. Local Coverage Determination (LCD): Controlled Substance Monitoring and Drugs of Abuse Testing(L36393). Centers for Medicare and Medicaid Services. Last revised January 17th 2018.https://www.cms.gov/medicare-coverage-database/details/lcd-details.aspx?LC-DId=36393&ver=24&Do- cID=L36393&bc=iAAAABAAAAAA&. Accessed on July 31, 2018.

11. Deborah Dowell, MD; Tamara M. Haegerich, Ph.D.; Roger Chou, MD. CDC Guideline for Prescribing Opioids for Chronic Pain. Morbidity and Mortality Weekly Report (MMWR). March 18, 2016. https://www.cdc.gov/ mmwr/volumes/65/rr/rr6501e1.htm. Accessed July 23, 2018.

Chapter 19

The Need for Prescribing Opioids

Opioids were initially designed to manage cancer pain, palliative care or end-of- life treatment, as well as postsurgical and severe acute pain. They have now become the essential elements in the management and treatment of all types of pain, and more specifically, chronic pain that is a noncancer-related pain.[1] Although controversial at the time, they have now found meaningful and productive uses in many areas of medicine. These include:

- Treating pain – chronic and acute
- Perioperative procedures – acute
- Cough suppressant
- Treatment of diarrhea.

Treating Pain – Chronic and Acute

The use of opioids to treat chronic back pain and acute illnesses become a more common practice in the early '80s to '90s. At that time, the pharmaceutical companies, medical associations, governmental agencies, and medical providers saw the opportunity to treat patients who were in pain chronically as well as acutely. There were significant marketing and promotional campaigns of opioids targeted at consumers, as well as physicians/providers and medical center medical centers or facilities.[2,3,4]

The treatment of pain always provides for challenging cases, even for seasoned professional pain management consultants.

Consider these four cases:

➢ **Patient: Mr. Leg, 25-year-old male**, who had a **broken leg** requiring surgery approximately two months ago. He has no complications from the surgery.

➢ **Patient: Ms. Norm, a 55-year-old housewife** with low back pain, has a normal MRI of her back.

➢ **Patient: Mr. Abnorm, a 70-year-old male**, has low back pain and neck pain and as an **abnormal MRI with multiple findings**. He had a **car accident** in his 20s; no significant injuries or surgeries.

➢ **Patient: Mr. Scar, a 55-year-old male**, has a **horrible looking** but healed **surgical scar** extending from his neck to his low back from multiple surgeries, the last one occurring **20 years ago.**

All patients have essentially normal exams except for some reported tenderness in areas that they were complaining about that were palpated.

The question is, who really has pain? Moreover, how do you tell who gets opioids and who does not, and how much? Sometimes, in some pain management practices, the decision is not always easy, and a lot of what is done in treating the patients relies not only on diagnostic studies and the patient's physical examination but also the patient's history as they present or as obtained by providers. Pain in and of itself is a subjective element, and each person experiences pain differently. Moreover, although there are many common characteristics or factors that help us as clinicians to determine the patients that genuinely need and deserve to be on opioids, the decision is not always easy.

We also have to bear in mind that patients generally present to offices for one of three primary reasons:

1. **They are in pain and believe treatment with or without opioids will be or may be helpful.** These are the vast majority of patients who have no specific agenda other than trying to get well.

2. **Patients who have some amount of pain, but have developed a tolerance or dependence on opioids**, and use opioids primarily because of the way it makes them feel, but not necessarily because their pain is significant. Most of these patients have been receiving opioids for a considerable length of time and have been treated in some instances with high doses. Although they are not the majority of pain patients, they form a significant group of patients who are prone to or are at higher risk for addiction.

3. **The dealers' group present to pain practices primarily to obtain opioids to sell, misuse and or abuse**. They themselves may not necessarily be addicted or have a tolerance or dependence on opioids.

These patients are presenting from all levels of economic, social, ethnic, racial and/or cultural types. A significant number of them have figured out how to navigate their way through pain management without being found out. Some of them will participate in procedures if it makes them appear more compliant.

They are definitely not the largest group of pain patients; however, they will form a significant part of the group from which opioids and other controlled substances diverge to users who are not necessarily patients under the care of healthcare providers.

The scenarios of patients above will often be treated differently, depending on each provider's approach. It is likely that in some practices, none of those patients may receive any opioids, or in others, all of them may receive them. This will be determined by the treating physicians/providers and their interpretations of the information that they have available to them in combination with the examination that they conducted.

The fact that someone has a large surgical scar or had surgery dating back to whenever does not necessarily mean that he or she is going to have pain. However, it also means that they are probably more likely to have it than someone who has never had surgery.

Abnormal MRI findings do not necessarily correlate with patients' pain. That is an abnormal finding is not equivalent to finding the source of one's pain. There are many individuals with abnormal imaging or MRI findings who have absolutely no pain. This does not mean they will or will not have in the future.

However, it is probably more likely that one will have pain that correlates with abnormal findings than if you have normal imaging studies. Similarly, patients with normal MRI does not exclude the possibility of them having pain.

The relevant questions then become: how do we treat these patients, and what other studies or consultants may be of help in the process of trying to find out the reasons for those apparent painful conditions?

The option of prescribing opioids may be limited to none in some practices. But there are patients who sometimes present to pain management practices on significant doses of opioids having similar scenarios.

In looking at treatments very often one of the questions for a pain management specialist who is evaluating a patient for the first time that is "taking" extremely large doses of opioids; is this patient taking all of these opioids? Sometimes, the answer is probably yes, but on numerous occasions, many of these patients will only use a portion of the medications that they were prescribed or receive, and the rest is diverted. In most of the instances where this occurs, patients are probably selling instead of giving away their medications. This is, of course, as opposed to family members who, without consent, lose their medications to diverters and/or other family members.

Despite the complexity and challenges involved in pain management, the treatment of pain is an indispensable part of medical care today in our society or any civilized society. This involves both chronic as well as acute pain.

The Treatment of Perioperative Pain

The treatment of perioperative pain is an essential part of minor and major surgical procedures. This allows, in the case of minor procedures, for patients to be more relaxed and tolerant of the procedures without the need for general anesthesia. In addition, a significant number of minor procedures is more effectively done with patients who are awake rather than when they are completely anesthetized and unable to communicate with the operating providers during the procedures.

There is no doubt that patients who underwent major surgical procedures benefit from opioids that are effective in treating severe pain.

Generally, this is given initially intravenously or via a **Patient-Controlled Analgesia pump** (PCA pump) during the course of their hospitalization, the patient will benefit immensely from oral opioids for moderate to severe pain postoperatively. In order to successfully perform most surgical procedures, particularly large surgeries, opioids are an essential part of the treatment protocols.

Without an adequate amount of intravenous opioids that can appropriately control patients' pain, most of these procedures will be drastically hampered or, in some instances, need to be cancelled. Patients typically undergoing these procedures will have moderate to severe pain that must be addressed at the end of the surgeries. Typically, medications such as intravenous fentanyl, Morphine, and Dilaudid are used and proven to be effective.

The FDA in November 2018 has approved an oral form of the drug **sufentanil.** Sold as **Dsuvia** and manufactured by AcelRx Pharmaceutical. **Sufentanil** is a synthetic opioid analog of fentanyl generally use intravenously to treat moderate to severe acute pain, and in epidurals. Dsuvia is about 10 times more potent than fentanyl. Fentanyl, on the other hand, is about 50 to 100 times more potent than morphine. It is expected that Dsuvia will be only available to be used in "certified healthcare facilities" and not sold or prescribed to the general public. Each tablet is expected to have a customized package (30 mcg). Dsuvia has sparked some controversy in part because of its potential for abuse as an opioid, its high potency, and its formulation as an oral tablet. However, the ease of use without the need for intravenous access has found significant support, particularly where such access is difficult to obtain or unavailable. [18,19]

The mobilization of patients (postoperatively in some instances) is extremely critical. Patients need to begin rehabilitation within 24 to 48 hours in some cases. Without adequate control of their pain, this would be virtually impossible. Opioids are also beneficial in the early acute phase of most major and some minor surgeries. In addition to surgeries, patients who have multiple traumas also benefit from opioids. This may also include patients who have suffered chemical or burn injuries, among others.

Non-Opioid Intravenous Perioperative Pain Medications

Although intravenous opioids are extremely effective in treating perioperative pain, there are alternatives. These include **intravenous acetaminophen (Ofirmev)**, **intravenous ketamine**,

Ketorolac IM/Intranasal, and **IV Liposomal Bupivacaine (Exparec)**. Numerous studies have shown the effectiveness of treating patients' perioperative pain with these medications.

Intravenous acetaminophen has been used successfully in treating pain in many surgical procedures such as joint replacement (where they are concluded in part: "These data suggest that intravenous acetaminophen is a useful component of the multimodal analgesia model, especially after major orthopedic surgery"), cardiac surgery (showed decrease in opioid consumption postoperatively), and gastrointestinal surgery, among others.

In 2014, gastric bypass surgery patients showed reduced pain with intravenous acetaminophen.[5,6,7]

The use of intravenous acetaminophen, however, is not without complaints or issues. Some studies have shown that it is not as good or effective as opioids. Also, there has been a noticeably dramatic increase in the price of some non- opioid alternative drugs for the treatment of acute pain that has made it financially challenging for hospitals/surgical centers and other acute facilities to justify their costs, including IV acetaminophen. Now although the cost of the IV formulation is significantly higher than the oral formulation, a controversial study has shown that there is not much difference in pain outcomes after open colectomy surgeries in patients who have taken oral versus IV medication, as reported in an article on *The Washington Post*. However, there is a greater number of studies and outcomes showing more beneficial effects of intravenous acetaminophen.[8,9]

Liposomal Bupivacaine is similarly used in pain management for surgery involving gynecology, total knee replacement, hemorrhoidectomy, and others.[10]

Other procedures involve orthopedic surgery such as joint replacements, gastrointestinal surgeries, and bariatric surgery (among others), resulting in the lowering of pain scores.[11]

It is also worth mentioning that studies have also shown that *one of the most frequent reasons for readmission following outpatient orthopedic procedures is inadequate pain control*. This result is up to 38% readmission. Also noted by another study is the inadequate pain treatment that postoperative patients often received. Hence, although these options are available, if not appropriately used, one can envision even higher readmissions to emergency rooms and/or hospitals for more adequate pain control.[12]

Also, in these scenarios, these patients were not necessarily on non-opioids, but were on opioids or treated with opioids perioperatively. Studies have also shown that up to 75% of patients in the United States are still not receiving appropriate postoperative pain control.[13,15]

Cough Suppressants

Opioids have also found use as suppressants in the treatment of cough and colds. **Dextromethorphan (DXM)**, an opioid, as well as **codeine and hydrocodone** are frequently found in cough medicine. **DXM** is often found in many over-the-counter medications, sometimes with or without antihistamines or decongestants.

It may be taken in liquid or pill form. There are numerous brands and configurations of cough medicines containing DXM. Although DXM is an opioid, it does not decrease pain. However, if the users dangerously consume significantly larger doses then medically recommended, users may experience an effect similar to those seen with hallucinogens like PCP and LSD. They may also experience effects similar to those associated with the intoxication of alcohol or marijuana, where depressant and/or hallucinogenic effects may be experienced, as well as some euphoria. These effects seen with DXM are varied and depend on many factors. Although they are significant, they are usually not at the same high or severe level associated with alcohol or the aforementioned drugs.

Cough medications containing codeine or hydrocodone are also significantly widely available and used to treat cough and colds. They also will have combinations of other medications, antihistamines, decongestants, etc. There are numerous combinations and brands available. Some of these medications are accessible only by prescription, while some of the codeine- containing cough medicines are available over-the-counter in some states.

In general, all these opioids containing medications and/or formulations of cough and cold medicines have the potential for abuse and misuse, and even a high probability of addiction developing from their inappropriate use. **The FDA now requires the labeling of prescriptions** for cough and cold medicine containing codeine and hydrocodone to be limited only to adults 18 years and older, as the risks outweigh the benefits for users less than 18 years old. It is recommended for those under 18 to be considered for non-opioid medications that have similar functions to those containing opioids but are safer for that age group. Cough and cold medicines containing DXM, although an opioid available over-the-counter, is also recommended, of course supervision and monitoring are imperative.[14]

Treatment for Diarrhea: Loperamide (Imodium)

Another significant area where opioids are used in treatment is diarrhea. **Loperamide (Imodium)** is an opioid that has found a use for the treatment of diarrhea. It may be in a pill or liquid form when taken. It may be present over- the-counter or by prescription. It works as an opioid agonist by attaching to receptors primarily outside of the brain (does not cross the blood-brain barrier).

It is not used to treat or relieve pain. It binds to the opioid receptors of the gut wall, resulting in the control or modification of diarrhea. It is also found to be useful in treating the gastrointestinal symptoms associated with opioid withdrawals. Some users do inappropriately frequently use high doses of loperamide to relieve withdrawal symptoms from opioids. This is not recommended and is dangerous; an overdose can cause the inability to urinate or urinary retention, an abnormal cardiac function that could lead to death, abnormal respiratory or breathing problems, the inability to move your bowels or severe constipation, severe nervous system problems, and many others. Always follow the instructions contained in the information package or leaflet that comes with the prescribed or over-the-counter medication.

In addition, detoxification from opioid withdrawals should be done only under medical supervision. It is important to realize that loperamide can be used and/or misused, and lead to addiction and/or overdose deaths.

The FDA has worked with manufacturers of **Loperamide** and other over-the-counter as well as prescription opioids to improve product safety by providing updated packaging information to enhance safety and compliance.

With all of these opioid medications, there is always the risk of use and abuse, as mentioned before. There are significant and ongoing attempts to create different concoctions or formulations using these medications. There is no limit to which this can be done. Moreover, although its practice is extremely dangerous, it is an active part of the opioid epidemic. There are users who sometimes use a wide range of illegal drugs such as cocaine or heroin or IMF to create whatever they think will be of benefit to them or meet their needs at that time. Unfortunately, this can often lead to fatal overdoses.[14]

The Other Side of Opioids

Most of this book has discussed what can go wrong when opioids are used both appropriately and inappropriately. This section in particular addresses the need for prescribing opioids; most of the negative consequences of the opioids have already been discussed in this book. However, I must also discuss the need to address another significant, less-talked-about side effect of opioids, commonly referred to as **Opioid-Induced Constipation (OIC);** this is the most common side effect for opioid users.[17]

Briefly, this is constipation related to the opioids binding to the receptors of the gastrointestinal tract (GI) and slowing down the activities of the GI tract, primarily bowel. Some companies have taken the initiative to develop and manufacture compounds specifically for opioid-induced constipation. Some examples are **Movantik (naloxegol)**, **Relistor (methylnaltrexone) and Symproic (naldemedine)**. They are μ-opioid receptor antagonists used to treat opioid-induced constipation in patients treated for chronic non-cancer pain.

In addition to compounds like these, in general, a good bowel program including but not limited to stool softeners, adequate hydration, and other non- opioid specific (Colace, Senokot, and MiraLAX, to name a few) medications are still very helpful and appropriate for use in most cases. And as always, just about every medication has side effects, and their use should be according to the manufacturers' and your healthcare providers' recommendations or instructions; and appropriate monitoring for side effects is always required.

References, Recommended Readings and Resources

1. Gery P. Guy Jr., Ph.D.; Kun Zhang, Ph.D.; Michele K. Bohm, MPH; Jan Losby, Ph.D.; Brian Lewis; Randall Young, MA; Louise B. Murphy, Ph.D.; Deborah Dowell, MD. CDCMMWR. Vital Signs: Changes in Opioid Pre- scribing in the United States, 2006–2015. July 7, 2017 / 66(26);697-704. https://www.cdc.gov/mmwr/volumes/66/wr/mm6626a4.htm?s_cid=m- m6626a4_w. Accessed March 1, 2018.

2. Department of Veterans Affairs, Pain as the Fifth Vital Sign Toolkit (October 2000) http://www.va.gov/PAINMANAGEMENT/docs/ TOOLKIT.pdf. Ac- cessed March 10, 2018.

3. Harvard Study: Big Pharma, US Gov. Behind Opioid Epidemic. July 27, 2017, Sean Adl-Tabatabai News, US 105. https://yournewswire. com/harvard-study-opioid-epidemic/. Accessed March 12, 2018.

4. Ritchie Farrell. The Opioid Epidemic: How Big Pharma and Congress Created America's Worst Health Crisis. 10/16/2017. https://www. huffington-post.com/entry/the-opioid-epidemic-how-big-pharma-and- congress-created_us_59e4e02ee4b003f928d5e8bf. Accessed March 7, 2018.

5. Shireesh Saurabh, M.D., Jessica K. Smith, M.D., Mark Pedersen, M.D., Paul Jose, M.D., Peter Nau, M.D., Isaac Samuel, M.D. Surgery for Obesity and Related Diseases Scheduled intravenous acetaminophen reduces postoperative narcotic analgesic demand and requirement after laparoscopic Roux-en-Y gastric bypass. September 23, 2014. https://www.soard.org/ article/S1550-7289(14)00357-8/ fulltext. Accessed July 7, 2018.

6. Srdjan Jelacic MD, Laurent Bollag MD, Andrew Bowdle MD, Ph.D., Cyril Rivat Ph.D., Kevin C. Cain Ph.D., Philippe Richebe MD, Ph.D. Journal of Cardiothoracic and Vascular Anesthesia Volume 30, Issue 4, August 2016, Pages 997-1004. Intravenous Acetaminophen as an Adjunct Analgesic in Cardiac Surgery Reduces Opioid Consumption but Not Opioid-Related Adverse Effects: A Randomized Controlled Trial. https://www.sciencedirect.com/science/article/pii/S1053077016000732. Last visited July 7, 2018.

7. Raymond S. Sinatra, M.D., Ph.D.; Jonathan S. Jahr, M.D.; Lowell W. Reynolds, M.D.; Eugene R. Viscusi, M.D.; Scott B. Groudine, M.D. Catherine Payen-Champenois, M.D. Anesthesiology 4 2005, Vol.102, 822-831. Efficacy and Safety of Single and Repeated Administration of 1 Gram Intravenous Acetaminophen Injection (Paracetamol) for Pain Management after Major Orthopedic Surgery. April 2005. http:// anesthesiology.pubs.asahq. org/Article.aspx?articleid=1941966. Accessed July 7, 2018.

8. Carolyn Y. Johnson. The growing case against IV Tylenol, once seen as a solution to the opioid crisis. June 19, 2018. https://www. washingtonpost. com/news/wonk/wp/2018/06/19/the-growing- case- against-iv-tylenol- once-seen-as-a-solution-to-the-opioid-crisis/?noredirect=on&utm_term=. e18979dba0b3. Accessed July 7, 2018.

9. Isaac Wasserman, M.P.H.; Jashvant Poeran, M.D., Ph.D.; Nicole Zubizarre- ta, M.P.H.; Jason Babby, Pharm.D., B.C.P.S.; Stelian Serban, M.D.; Andrew T. Goldberg, M.D.; Alexander J. Greenstein, M.D.; Stavros G. Memtsoudis, M.D., Ph.D.; Madhu Mazumdar, Ph.D.; Andrew Leibowitz, M.D. Impact of Intravenous Acetaminophen on Perioperative Opioid Utilization and Outcomes in Open Colectomies: A Claims Database Analysis. Anesthesiology 7 2018, Vol.129, 77-88. July 2018. http://anesthesiology.pubs.asahq.org/article.aspx?articleid=2679411. Accessed June 21, 2018.

10. Bryan Sakamoto, MD, Ph.D.; Shelly Keiser, PharmD; Russell Meldrum, MD; Gene Harker, MD, Ph.D.; Andrew Freese, MD. JAMA Surg. 2017;152(1):90-95. Efficacy of Liposomal Bupivacaine Infiltration on the Management of Total Knee Arthroplasty. January 2017. https://jamanetwork.com/journals/jamasurgery/fullarticle/2566221. Accessed July 7, 2018.

11. Stokes, Audrey L. M.D.; Adhikary, Sanjib D. M.D.; Quintili, Ashley Pharm.D.; Puleo, Frances J. M.D.; Choi, Christine S. M.D.; Hollenbeak, Christopher S. Ph.D.; Messaris, Evangelos M.D., Ph.D. Liposomal Bupivacaine Use in Transversus Abdominis Plane Blocks Reduces Pain and Postoperative Intravenous Opioid Requirement After Colorectal Surgery. Diseases of the Colon & Rectum: February 2017 - Volume 60 - Issue 2- p 170–177. https://journals.lww.com/dcrjournal/Abstract/2017/02000/Liposomal_Bupivacaine_Use_in_ Transversus_Abdominis.7.aspx. Accessed July 7, 2018.

12. Coley KC, Williams BA, DaPos SV, Chen C, Smith RB Retrospective evaluation of unanticipated admissions and readmissions after same-day surgery and associated costs. J Clin Anesth. 2002 Aug;14(5):349-53. https:// www.ncbi.nlm.nih.gov/ pubmed/12208439. Last visited August 4, 2018.

13. Wu CL, Raja SN. Treatment of acute postoperative pain. Lancet. 2011 Jun 25;377(9784):2215-25. https://www.ncbi.nlm.nih.gov/ pubmed/21704871. Last visited August 4, 2018.

14. NIH. National Institute of drug abuse. Commonly abused drugscharts. January 2018. https://www.drugabuse.gov/drugs-abuse/commonly- abused- drugs-charts. Accessed July 7, 2018.

15. Donald M. Phillips. JCAHO Pain Management Standards Are Unveiled. JAMA. 2000;284(4):428-429. July 26, 2000. https:// jamanetwork.com/ journals/jama/article-abstract/2552036. Last visited August 4, 2018.

16. Deborah Dowell, MD; Tamara M. Haegerich, Ph.D.; Roger Chou, MD. CDC Guideline for Prescribing Opioids for Chronic Pain. Morbidity and Mortality Weekly Report (MMWR). March 18, 2016. https://www.cdc.gov/mmwr/volumes/65/rr/rr6501e1.htm. Accessed July 23, 2018.

17. S.J. Panchal, P. Müller-Schwefe, J.I. Wurzelmann. Opioid-induced bowel dysfunction: prevalence, pathophysiology and burden. 04 May 2007. https://onlinelibrary.wiley.com/doi/full/10.1111/j.1742-1241.2007.01415.x Access July 22, 2018.

18. Abby Goodnough. The New York Times. F.D.A. Approves Powerful New Opioid Despite Warnings of Likely Abuse. Nov. 2, 2018 https://www.nytimes.com/2018/11/02/health/dsuvia-fda-opoid.html Last accessed November 5, 2018

19. Shelia M. Poole. The Atlanta Journal-Constitution, Powerful new drug Dsuvia sparks fears amid opioid epidemic. Nov 4, 2018. https://www.kiro7.com/news/trending-now/powerful-new-drug-dsuvia-sparks-fears-amid-opioid-epidemic/866230193 Last accessed November 5, 2018.

Chapter 20

Do Not Let our Pain Patients Suffer –
This May Be You Someday

There are indeed some undeniable truths about the opioid epidemic. Here are a few of them:

➢ The opioid epidemic is real.[1]
➢ Medical doctors and healthcare providers contributed to the cause of the opioid epidemic. Pain doctors are responsible for less than six percent (6%) of all opioid prescriptions filled in the United States.[2]
➢ Pharmaceutical companies contributed to the cause of the opioid epidemic.[3,4]
➢ The government and politicians contribute to the cause of the opioid epidemic.[3,4,5]
➢ Illegal opioids are responsible for more opioid deaths than legally prescribed opioids by far.[6,7]
➢ The number of opioid deaths continues to increase in spite of legally prescribed opioids continuing to decrease since 2010.[7]
➢ Illegal drugs like cocaine, methamphetamine and non-opioid drugs killed more people than legally prescribed opioids.[6]
➢ The opioid epidemic requires collaborative efforts from multiple sources, including the medical and political communities, law enforcement, social and community service organizations, pharmaceutical companies, and healthcare insurance providers, to name a few.
➢ We can all do more, and we all must do more to reverse and control the opioid epidemic.

➤ The government, politicians, state and federal agencies can create as many laws, rules and regulations as they see they fit. They may even send as many doctors or providers and drug dealers to jail for as long as they choose. However, they cannot legislate away people's real pain, the vast majority of whom are good and law-abiding people who simply need help.

Let me elaborate on the opioid epidemic that in part concerns legally prescribed opioids. More than 115 people are dying each day from opioid-related deaths. This includes both legal, and illegal drugs such as heroin and IMF. About 40% of all opioid deaths are attributed to legally prescribed opioids; which therefore implies that legally prescribed opioids are responsible for about 46 deaths per day, or that about one person dies each day in every state in the United States, on average. Now, of course, it would be an amazing accomplishment if no one ever died from an opioid-related prescription drug in our state each day. [1,6,8]

If you look at the short list of 10 truths above, I hope that you agree that we shouldn't take this opioid epidemic for granted. However, I must also ask how many people die each day on average in our respective states from car accidents, gun-related incidents, and alcohol-related incidents. and you can choose whichever categories make you feel most comfortable or uncomfortable, for that matter[2,10,11]

Once you're finished analyzing the number of deaths in the categories of your choice, the question is then: do you remove or limit the use of the objects that cause deaths in those categories? You would also notice that overdose deaths from prescription opioids are at least 50% less in any of those categories.

The point is, as important as the opioid epidemic is, it is also important that we do not needlessly overreact and cause the suffering of a large number of patients that truly need and deserve to be on opioids responsibly.

Also, we must brace ourselves for an increasing need for pain management for an aging population that will comprise a larger percentage of seniors in the near future than we have today. Opioids use must be monitored appropriately, and prescriptions should be given and dispensed according to appropriate guidelines and by professionals who understand and can ensure that patients are appropriately treated with the medications and services that they deserve. You will notice in this book that I firmly believe, like so many practicing pain management physicians and providers, that opioids, as important as they are, are just one of many tools that we utilize in the management of pain. But opioids are extremely important tools used not just for treating chronic pain but also for acute pain.

Many perioperative procedure-related conditions and non-operative related injuries have relied on opioids for successful outcomes.

Many patients have significant fears about using opioids because of the potential risk of addiction. These fears are justified to some degree. However, the reality is that most patients who are treated with opioids and use them appropriately never become addicted or dependent on them. According to the CDC, about 8% to 12% of opioid users are likely to become addicted or develop a dependence on opioids.[12]

Most patients who are using opioids appropriately have the potential to stop or transition to other treatments that will allow them to have better control of their pain. *It is so crucial that chronic pain patients are not stigmatized as drug addicts or people who are incapable of managing their lives or illness as it relates to substance abuse and psychosocial issues.*

Chronic pain, as well as acute pain, is real, even though there are a significant number of patients and individuals who abuse opioids as well as controlled substances for almost everything except pain. It is up to the professionals who treat these patients to make the distinctions and address those issues accordingly. Of course, all patients need to be monitored appropriately and treated according to their medical needs.[19] We truly hope, as physicians and healthcare providers, that we will continue to make those decisions with our patients; rather than allowing politicians and healthcare insurance providers to do so.

We all can agree that the opioid epidemic is real, and the deaths from opioid overdose keep increasing despite the efforts being made to curtail this crisis. However, it is also worth noting that although non-opioids are in part the answer to some of the problems, we must bear in mind that medications such as **acetaminophen (Tylenol)** is the primary cause of **liver failure and associated deaths** in our country. Also, **gastrointestinal and kidney disorders and associated cardiac deaths** as well as other significant complications from **nonsteroidal anti-inflammatory drugs (NSAIDs)** such as ibuprofen and naproxen, which are commonly used, and cannot and should not go unnoticed.

An article titled Deadly NSAIDs published by the American Nutrition Association in part described the devastating effect of NSAIDs. This article also referred to a statement from a July 1998 issue of The American Journal of Medicine in which at least 16,500 people are believed to die each year from related complications of NSAIDs.[24] Now, this number of deaths is more than that associated with legally prescribed opioids and is a significant number when compared with illegal opioids depending on time frame of comparison.

It is reasonable to say that all medications carry potential risks of varying degrees. Patients' appropriate usage of and adherence to the instructions that accompany the medications, regardless of whether they are opioids or non- opioids, are critical elements that must be part of their care.

Many publications are available that have shown that one of the most significant reasons for **postsurgical readmissions** to emergency rooms or hospitals is poor pain control. That is, not the surgeries or complications from them, but simply uncontrollable or intolerable pain. Ironically, some of these publications were available well before alternative treatments began to be used, such as intravenous acetaminophen and other non-opioids, now more common than in the past. This leads some experts in the field of pain management to believe that if opioids, as potent as they are, are unable to control acute pain effectively, then how much can we rely on acetaminophen and some of the others as realistic alternative options? This does not mean of course that alternative treatments should not be sought and or utilized.[21,22]

The DEA in 2017 has reduced the quota of opioids produced by 25% of was produce in the year 2016. is expected in 2018 to reduce the resulting manufactured volume of 2017 by about 20%, and in the year 2019, by 10%.

This has resulted in a tremendous shortage in many pharmacies, particularly smaller pharmacies and those in rural areas. Therefore, some patients have more difficulties obtaining the prescriptions that they need. These reductions sometimes require them to go to multiple pharmacies at a greater distance in order to complete their prescriptions. [20,23]

Although most of these other small pharmacies are dispensing and monitoring opioids and other controlled substances appropriately and abiding by the rules, regulations, and laws in place, some do not follow appropriately. Patients using multiple pharmacies sometimes can and often lead to increasing diversions, among other misuse. This does not eliminate the same problems from also happening in the larger, more established pharmacies. However, there should be a balance in how the reduction of opioid manufacture and the needs of patients for legitimate prescriptions of opioids are approached.

The other scenarios that are often met with great difficulties and challenges are the limited availability of IV opioids typically used in surgical settings because of the DEA's decision to reduce opioid production.[20] This has affected surgical procedures being performed, as well as postoperative treatments. The shortage of opioids is also affecting the rehabilitation of patients who need to be functional in acute settings before being discharged to a lower level of care or home.

The other major factor that is often a challenge for all of us who prescribe opioids and those of us responsible in part for their appropriate use in treating patients who are no longer receiving opioids or cannot afford the costs of opioids. These patients resort to what they believed to be a substitute for the prescription drugs that there were taking, only to be pulled into the illegal world of heroin, IMF as well as other synthetic analogs. These drugs are generally much cheaper, deadlier, more addictive. In addition, they are often associated with criminal activities such as and trafficking.[7,8]

When we tried to assess the beginning of the opioid epidemic, many people will point to certain events in time and say this was when it started. However, looking as far back as we want to look, it is reasonable to say we have always had a drug problem. We may not have looked at it the way that we do today, and statistics may not have been as accessible as they are today, and neither were they analyzed as they are now.

Some of us will look at events like the beginning and the use of "pain as the fifth vital sign" by the Department of Veterans Affairs, supported by the vast majority of credible medical associations and many experts in the field of pain management at that time, and say that that was a major contravening factor or a turning point.[5]

Today, there are those who question the need for a fifth vital sign. I'm one of those who believe that it is still an important part of addressing patients' needs during their periods of illnesses and recovery, particularly those patients who are likely to have pain. There are so many patients admitted because of trauma and multiple related injuries, as well as those who have undergone elective and necessary surgical procedures in some cases to improve the quality of their lives, functional status and need to reduce the amount of pain that they were experiencing. There are some experts and some non-experts out there who will tell you that the fifth vital sign is not important and should be disregarded. However, for those patients who have had tremendous injuries and have had surgeries, pain control is a critically important aspect of their recovery.

For those of us who work in pain management and acute hospital settings, where we are entrusted to take care of patients who have undergone or had significant illness resulting in pain, we can assure you there is no other rational way but to treat their pain. We often would not accomplish much if we require someone to get moving after they have had their knee or hip replaced, back surgeries, or abdominal surgeries and expect them to walk with minimal pain control.

It is very important that patients be mobilized and up and out of bed soon after their surgeries are completed, as long as their conditions allow them to tolerate the level of activity that they will encounter during the initial phase of **Acute Rehabilitation.** If the patients are unable to get up and out of bed because their pain is unsatisfactorily controlled, the risks of catastrophic and sometimes fatal complications are significantly increased. In addition, patients' long-term recovery is made even longer without appropriate rehabilitation soon after surgeries.

Also, a critical point is; the presence or absence of pain provides the clinicians often with helpful insights into other aspects of patients' clinical/medical status just as much as blood pressure, heart rate, temperature, and respiration rate do. The importance of each vital sign will depend on the correlation it has with each patient's medical condition at the time of evaluation.

Hopefully, we will not go back to the days when patients sued their doctors for not properly taking care of their pain, as they did in California. Neither should we go back to the days when medical boards were disciplining doctors because they failed to take care of their patients' pain needs adequately.[13,14]

Rational thinking and approach to this complex problem are not easy, but it is achievable. So often in our society, there are knee-jerk reactions to many problems without considering the long-term or even the short-term consequences. Hopefully, as important as the opioid epidemic is, we as professionals, as well as people in all sectors of our society who have a vested interest in taking care of others, we will not fall short, resulting in increasing the suffering of patients. If we fail to manage their pain appropriately, our patients will become less functional thereby experiencing more pain.[17,18]

References, Recommended Readings and Resources

1. Center for Disease Control and Prevention. Understanding the Epidemic. https://www.cdc.gov/drugoverdose/epidemic/index.html. Last visited June 16, 2018.
2. Levy B, Paulozzi L, Mack KA, Jones CM. Trends in Opioid Analgesic- Prescribing Rates by Specialty, U.S., 2007-2012. Am J Prev Med. 2015 Sep;49(3):409-13. Apr 18, 2015.Opioid Overdose Prescribing Data. https://www.cdc.gov/drugoverdose/data/prescribing. html. Accessed May 26, 2018.
3. Harvard Study: Big Pharma, US Gov. Behind Opioid Epidemic. July 27, 2017, Sean Adl-Tabatabai News, US 105. https://yournewswire. com/harvard-study-opioid-epidemic/. Accessed March 12,2018.

4. Ritchie Farrell. The Opioid Epidemic: How Big Pharma and Congress Created America's Worst Health Crisis. 10/16/2017. https://www. huffington-post.com/entry/the-opioid-epidemic-how-big-pharma-and- congress-created_us_59e4e02ee4b003f928d5e8bf. Accessed March 7, 2018.

5. Department of Veterans Affairs, Pain as the Fifth Vital Sign Toolkit (October 2000). http://www.va.gov/PAINMANAGEMENT/docs/ TOOLKIT.pdf. Accessed March 10, 2018.

6. Gery P. Guy Jr., Ph.D.; Kun Zhang, Ph.D.; Michele K. Bohm, MPH; Jan Losby, Ph.D.; Brian Lewis; Randall Young, MA; Louise B. Murphy, Ph.D.; Deborah Dowell, MD. CDCMMWR. Vital Signs: Changes in Opioid Pre- scribing in the United States, 2006–2015. July 7, 2017 / 66(26);697-704. https://www.cdc.gov/mmwr/volumes/66/wr/ mm6626a4.htm?s_cid=m- m6626a4_w. Accessed March 1, 2018.

7. U.S. drug overdose deaths continue to rise; increase fueled by synthetic opioids. https://www.cdc.gov/media/releases/2018/p0329- drug-overdose- deaths.html. Accessed May 5, 2018.

8. Puja Seth, Ph.D.; Lawrence Scholl, Ph.D.; Rose A. Rudd, MSPH; Sarah Bacon, Ph.D., MMMWR. Overdose deaths involving opioids, cocaine, and psychostimulants – United States, 2015 – 2016. https:// www.cdc.gov/ mmwr/volumes/67/wr/mm6712a1.htm. Accessed May 5, 2018.

9. Motor vehicle fatality rate in U.S. by year. https://en.wikipedia.org/ wiki/ Motor_vehicle_fatality_rate_in_U.S._by_year. Accessed July 16, 2018.

10. Jennifer Mascia. 15 Statistics That Tell the Story of Gun Violence in 2015. December 23, 2015. https://www.thetrace.org/2015/12/gun- violence-stats-2015/. Accessed July 16, 2018.

11. Centers for Disease Control and Prevention (CDC). Fact Sheets - Alcohol Use and Your Health. Atlanta, GA: CDC. https://www.cdc. gov/alcohol/ fact-sheets/alcohol-use.htm. Last visited July 22, 2018.

12. NIH. National Institute on Drug Abuse. Opioid overdose crisis. https:// www.drugabuse.gov/drugs-abuse/opioids/opioid-overdose-crisis. Ac- cessed June 4, 2018.

13. Oregon Board Disciplines Doctor for Not Treating Patients' Pain," New York Times, September 4, 1999, http://www.nytimes. com/1999/09/04/us/oregon-board-disciplines-doctor-for-not-treating- patients-pain.html. Accessed March 10, 2018

14. Bergman v. Eden Medical Center, No. H205732-1 (Cal.Super. Ct., Alameda County, 2001). https://www.highbeam.com/ doc/1G1-79341880.html. Ac- cessed March 10, 2018

15. Furrow, B. R. "Pain Management and Provider Liability: No More Excuses" Journal of Law, Medicine & Ethics 29, no. 1(2001): 28– 51, SAGEJournals.http://journals.sagepub.com/doi/10.1111/j.1748- 720X.2001. tb00038.x. Accessed March 10, 2018.

16. Perry G Fine, West J Med. Fear and Loathing on the Care Path Treating Pain and Suffering. 2002 Jan; 176(1):17. https://www.ncbi. nlm.nih.gov/pmc/articles/PMC1071643/. Accessed March 10, 2018

17. Rick Lunkenheimer. HuffPost. There's Another Opioid Crisis We Don't Talk About and I'm Trapped in The Middle of It. July 5, 2018. https:// www.huffingtonpost.com/entry/opioid-crisis-chronic- pain_ us_5b3a4e- b2e4b09e4a8b25ebe6. Last visited July 14, 2018.

18. Sarah Vander Schaaff. The Washington Post. Amid the opioid crisis, some seriously ill people risk losing drugs they depend on. July 14, 2018. https://www.washingtonpost.com/national/health-science/amid-the-opi- oid-crisis- some-seriously-ill-people-risk-losing-drugs-they-depend- on/2018/07/13/65850640- 730d-11e8-805c-4b67019fcfe4_ story.html?utm_term=.8b404f003e89. Accessed July 14, 2018

19. Deborah Dowell, MD; Tamara M. Haegerich, Ph.D.; Roger Chou, MD. CDC Guideline for Prescribing Opioids for Chronic Pain. Morbidity and Mortality Weekly Report (MMWR). March 18, 2016. https://www.cdc.gov/ mmwr/volumes/65/rr/rr6501e1.htm. Accessed July 23, 2018.

20. Robert W. Patterson. Statement Before the House Judiciary Committee U.S. House of Representatives For a Hearing Entitled: "Challenges and Solutions in the Opioid Abuse Crisis" Presented on May 08, 2018 https:// www.dea.gov/pr/speeches- testimony/2018t/050818t.pdf. Last visited August 1 18.

21. Coley KC, Williams BA, DaPos SV, Chen C, Smith RB Retrospective evaluation of unanticipated admissions and readmissions after same day surgery and associated costs. J Clin Anesth. 2002 Aug;14(5):349-53. https:// www.ncbi.nlm.nih.gov/ pubmed/12208439. Last visited August 4, 2018.

22. Wu CL, Raja SN. Treatment of acute postoperative pain. Lancet. 2011 Jun 25;377(9784):2215-25. https://www.ncbi.nlm.nih.gov/ pubmed/21704871. Last visited August 4, 2018.

23. Justice Department, DEA Propose Significant Opioid Manufacturing Reduction in 2019. August 16, 2018. https://www.justice.gov/opa/pr/ justice-de- partment-dea- propose-significant-opioid-manufacturing- reduction-2019. Last visited August 21, 2018.

24. Deadly NSAIDs. American Nutrition Association. http:// americannutritionassociation.org/newsletter/deadly-nsaids Accessed October 26, 2018.

Chapter 21

What about Law Enforcement, Healthcare Insurance Companies, Politics, and Money?

In the initial stage of planning and writing this book, I decided that I would have at least a chapter each for law enforcement, health insurance companies, politics, and who is paying for all of this stuff – finances. As I've learned more about the subject of the opioid epidemic and the various components and parts that are essential in dealing with this problem, I have decided simply to stick with medicine. The primary reason is this: any of these topics will simply overwhelm and suppress the importance of what this book is about and its subject matter: the opioid epidemic.

The issues surrounding these four areas are extremely complex, of critical importance, and requires an in-depth and comprehensive approach for each sector to play the essential role it has. I have decided that those areas are beyond the scope of this book, as important as they are. Each of these areas represents a subject matter with far more information to complete more than a book for each category. The occasional comments on each area throughout this book does not in part constitute the appropriate level of discussion or commentary necessary for you to be informed consumers or providers capable of making a rational conclusion from this book about these sectors.

Conclusion

My Parting Thoughts

The opioid epidemic is one of the most significant crises this country has ever faced. It is a problem that has multiple dimensions. It is not just a national health or medical crisis; a law enforcement issue; a political problem; an economic burden; or a social, racial or cultural problem. It is all these things combined to form one of our greatest human catastrophes.

It is not uncommon in times like these to hear people say: "This does not affect me; it is probably not real, so who cares? I have nothing to do with it." 'Those people' are the problem. However, if you can accept the premise that we all have a problem that is very complex and multidimensional, you can be a part of the solution that will require inputs from many different sources for an extended period. The opioid epidemic is real; and just like all the other drugs or substance abuse issues, unfortunately, it is not getting better soon. The opioid epidemic will evolve; we all hope it can and will change for the better. But one of the sad truths is that it has a significant potential to get even worse.

You have read this book. I am sure that you realize the information that I used in part to understand this opioid epidemic is driven by statistical data. The way data were collected, and statistics were compiled and analyzed, as well as the large volume of information that will have to be processed, have left us literally chasing numbers as we watch the figures for opioid-overdose deaths continue to rise. In 2018, we are looking at data and figures primarily from 2015 and 2016, with information for 2017 yet to be fully available.

In August 2018, the NIH published an article indicating that the projected or estimated total deaths from drug overdose in 2017 will exceed 72,000.

The number of deaths from illegal opioids, primarily IMF and its analogs, are expected to be about 30,000. This is the nature of the data collection process; it is not a reflection of the numerous people working diligently to provide the information that we desperately need.

What Do We Know from All the Data We Have Collected?

Medical Doctors and Providers' Role

Medical doctors or healthcare providers are considered among the main contributors to the cause of the opioid epidemic. While this has some truth to it, the actual number of prescriber-related opioid deaths is about 25% of all drug- associated deaths.

It is also worth noting that pain doctors or pain management specialists do not contribute significantly to the opioid epidemic, by virtue of the fact that the total number of prescriptions from us is less than six (6) percent of all opioids prescribed in the United States.

It is essential to understand the critical role that not only pain management physicians and their providers can play in the opioid epidemic, but also other physicians and their medical providers who are trained and have ascertained relevant knowledge not only to prescribe responsibly but also offer additional treatments other than opioids.

Sometimes, We're Not as Good as They Say We Are

In most instances, the patient-doctor relationship is very good. It is not uncommon for patients to say wonderful things about their doctors, recommend other patients to their practices, even travel far distances to see them and, in some instances, bring gifts. However, for pain management and other doctors who write prescriptions for opioids and other controlled substances, this relationship may be different. These doctors sometimes have to be cynical about those patients who praise them and pretended to do all the right things.

It doesn't matter how good you are as physicians or providers. It is unlikely that patients in the ordinary course of their daily life will travel across state lines or travel great distant just to be treated in order to get opioids and controlled substances.

In addition, even for those of us who do procedures for pain management, we are just not that hard to find, and no one should have the need to travel hours to get to us or go across various state lines for the special services that we offer at our practices. Whenever these patients present themselves to us, it should be at the very least a "yellow flag." Either the patients, the providers or both are probably doing something not commonly done by most other patients or providers, whether the providers are aware of it or not. Most people don't want to travel even an hour to get to their doctors unless there are some unique or different specialties or procedures that are not readily available in their local areas.

The VIPs

Sometimes, in an effort to be friendly and non-confrontational, there are some physicians and providers who will simply not follow the protocols that are consistent with the standard of care when treating their colleagues, colleagues' families, CEO of the of the hospital, and other "important people." These providers fail to do the same testing such as urine drug testing for illicit drugs, alcohol, and medication compliance that everyone of their "normal patients" goes through. This failure to follow protocols could lead to drug abuse and even deaths, as is often implied in the deaths of some famous people who were not required to follow the same guidelines as everyone else.

Willful Ignorance

Some physicians and providers indulge in what is best described as "willfulignorance." This is described by Definition.net as:

A bad faith decision to avoid becoming informed about something to avoid having to make undesirable decisions that such information might prompt. It may also be shown as for a person to have no clue in a decision but still goes ahead in their decision.[1]

One example might be someone who knows the symptoms of colon cancer and is experiencing what appears to be consistent with them. However, that person refused to do any testing to find out whether or not the cancer is present. This is an effort to avoid facing the consequences of possibly having colon cancer.

Another example is; some physicians or providers who strongly suspect or are aware of patients using marijuana, but decide not to test for it. They feel justified in continuing to write prescriptions for opioids and other controlled substances because they have "no knowledge of their patients' marijuana use." Marijuana is used in this case, but willful ignorance is also applicable to other controlled, illegal substances or even legal substances such as alcohol.

A caregiver with chronic pain takes her disabled adult child to a pain management doctor care doctor stating that he had an insignificant fall with no specific injury and had been in pain. Both the caregiver and the child have been on high-dose opioids for years and stated that their primary care physician continues to treat them for pain. Moreover, the primary care sees them about every two weeks for a long time.

Among the questions, of course, is: does the provider really believe that the disabled or impaired patient is receiving and ingesting all the high-dose opioids provided, or are they being diverted? Moreover, how long will it take before the primary care provider stop and realize that their action is not helpful?

Does he or she simply continue to treat those patients, even though it is more probable that the caregiver may be doing something wrong?

In September 2018, the news media carried a news story regarding a medical doctor, Barry Schultz, who was sentenced in Florida to 157 years in prison for his role in overprescribing opioids. This article reported that for a period of about eight months, DEA records indicated that one patient was prescribed more than 23,000 high-dose oxycodone pills, presumably to treat his or her specific painful condition. Now, this is about 100 pills per day; let's assume that the authorities holding him responsible is off by about 50%. That leaves about 50 opioid pills for one patient to take each day.

The obvious and simple question is: how does any patient take that much medications? Moreover, if he or she did that, how would that patient survive and live to do it all over again the next day?

As a consumer or a medical provider, you could ask yourself a myriad of questions without finding any rational answers. This is in part what willful ignorance can do to those who indulge in it.[4]

Your Patient is Nice

Your patient is nice and is a decent and kind person. But don't let this fool you. Some of these patients who will frequently abuse and misuse opioids and controlled substances have some of the best interpersonal skills. Maybe it is required as part of negotiating drug use in the community or the environment they are from. These patients should always be monitored very closely. Again, it is not always wrong to be cynical.

Cash for Services Rendered

There is nothing wrong with any patients presenting at a medical facility and paying cash for the medical service provided. In fact, in our society cash is important because a significant number of patients that have no healthcare insurance and sometimes paying cash to the healthcare providers is much cheaper than paying high healthcare insurance premiums.

Some of these insurance policies have very limited benefits unless there is a catastrophic or significant medical illness. Generally, deductibles are extremely high, and a considerable number of patients who do not have any significant illness is unlikely to meet their deductibles. However, sometimes we are seeing what many believe to have been the genesis of the opioid epidemic, when the **Pill mills** were created: fast cash for limited and often inappropriate service, with patients getting virtually what they want regarding high-dose and large quantities of opioids as well as controlled substances. Very often, anyone who is paying cash for anything believes that they should dictate what they receive for their money. In the case of physicians/providers who are unable to function without money dictating what they do or how they practice, the cash-for-service practice has the potential for worsening the opioid epidemic.

It is important to note that the amount of money you can afford to pay should not dictate and cannot dictate the type or the quantity of opioids or controlled substances that you receive as patients. Neither should the kind of healthcare insurance that you have, nor "high" or "indigent" status in society dictate the care you received.

In most pain management practices, the costs for office visits and laboratory studies often make most cash- paying patients less likely to seek services from our facilities; it is simply too expensive.

Moving Forward

The Human Health Services Acting Secretary declared a Public Health Emergency to Address National Opioid Crisis in October 2017.

This statement in October 2017 was well crafted and probably represents where the administration believes we are in terms of the opioid epidemic based on whatever information they are looking at. However, I can't help wondering that the statement should have been:

The Human Health Services Acting Secretary declared a National Opioid Epidemic Emergency to Address a Public Health Crisis in October 2017

At what point do we go from looking at the budget of the Department of Health and Human Services, and instead providing a separate and special budge to address the opioid health crisis thus making funding available to combat the opioid epidemic. Clearly, to many experts in the field of pain management and addiction medicine the opioid epidemic a national emergency involving all of America.

In 2016, we had over 63,000 people dying from a drug overdose, 42,000 of which were opioid-related. It is projected that in 2017, the total number is expected to exceed 72,000 drug overdose-related deaths.[3]

The questions are: is 100,000, 120,000, or 150,000 the more appropriate number before we get to a national emergency, and when will we be there? Alternatively, does the government simply believe that we have reached the maximum number of opioid deaths that we will ever have? Of course, my wish is that we never get close to 100,000 deaths, but as we look at all the indicators and what is being done, I would be pleasantly surprised if we are not over 100,000 by the end of the year 2019. Unfortunately, we will not know this until the year 2020 or 2021.

I genuinely hope I'm wrong about this, because as we are now, the impact of the opioid epidemic is extremely devastating, to say the least. Moreover, if you are still asking what the difference between those two declarations is, it is simply a matter of utilization of resources and where to use funds where they are most needed. The appropriate allocation of funds can make an enormous difference in the path the opioid epidemic will take.

In Closing, here are 10 Things We Must Keep in Mind
(Of Course, Numerous Others Can be Found Throughout this Book)

1. **Naloxone** still remains the most significant medication in the fight against the opioid epidemic regarding saving lives.

2. **Illegal opioids** such as IMF and its analogs are responsible for more opioid deaths than legally prescribed opioids as well as non-opioid drugs. This category is the fastest growing and deadliest category to be dealt with if the opioid epidemic is to be contained. The others, of course, should not be ignored.

3. **The number of opioid deaths continues to increase, although the number of legally prescribed opioids continue to decrease since 2010.** There needs to be a paradigm shift inasmuch as there need to be improvements in all categories, primarily with doctors and providers. The Pill mills are almost gone, and the diversion of opioids and other controlled substances is declining. It is only a matter of time that the effort spent in this category although still necessary will yield very little to decrease the rise in the number of opioid deaths.

4. **Illegal drugs like cocaine, methamphetamine and non-opioid drugs killed more people than legally prescribed opioids.** The focus on the opioid epidemic seems to have left this category with a free pass. This category continues to be dangerous, not only because some of the illegal drugs are used in combination with illicit opioids, but because this group also continues to grow and a significant number of deaths are resulting from this group, second only to illegal opioids.

5. **The opioid epidemic requires collaborative efforts from multiple sources**, including medical, political, law enforcement, social and community service organizations, pharmaceutical companies, and healthcare insurance provider. The blame game or who gets credit should be secondary to the need for all entities to work together for one common goal. This is the minimum requirement in order to control the opioid epidemic.

6. **Education has always been the cornerstone of most successful entities and processes**. The opioid epidemic is one which requires extensive educational efforts to improve awareness, treatment, support among the different organizations and services, and access, particularly for those who may be unaware or unable to obtain needed help because of multiple factors. We all can do more, and we all must do more to reverse and control the opioid epidemic. Not only politicians, law enforcement, healthcare providers, and services, but everyone needs to do their part.

7. **The government, pharmaceutical companies, ancillary service providers, healthcare service providers and healthcare insurance companies have to find a collaborative way** to make the medications, services, and processes required to control this epidemic affordable, particularly for those who are more likely to be adversely affected but are financially incapable of benefiting because of the lack of funds.

8. **The use of alternative or complementary/non-traditional medicine and traditional medicine/modern medicine should be supported** because they aid in the prevention and reduction of the need for opioids and other controlled substances.

9. **Physicians and healthcare providers are responsible in part** and are held accountable for the opioid epidemic. Similarly, **government and state agencies have a responsibility to hold healthcare insurance companies, as well as pharmaceutical companies, responsible for the role they are playing**, or are failing to play in this opioid epidemic.

10. **The government, politicians, state and federal agencies** can create as many laws, rules, and regulations as they see fit. They may even send as many doctors or providers and drug dealers to jail for as long as they choose. However, they **cannot legislate away people's pain:** that is real. The vast majority of pain patients are good law-abiding people who simply need help. It is essential that a responsible and rational approach be taken to the use of opioids and controlled substances for everyone who prescribes, particular those of us who are at the front and center of this epidemic in whatever capacity.

The Opioid Epidemic is Real
as Are the People and their Life Stories

I have stated in this book that the information contained herein is not a reflection of our practice or how anyone in particular that I know practice, and that remained so throughout the book. However, I will share two of my patients' stories with you in closing. Some of the information has been modified to protect the identity of the patients and their healthcare confidentiality.

Mary Jane is a 68-year-old female who presents for pain management. She has been in and out of pain management and presented at our office for the management of her chronic pain. She appears reasonably credible after reviewing all available documentation and completing her history and physical examination, as well as reviewing all available medical records.

Notable in her patient social history is that she had lost a daughter about two years ago, whom she described as having died from heroin laced with IMF. Her daughter was a heroin addict. She also stated that about three months ago, she lost her second son who was murdered for unknown reasons. These were "her two best children," she stated; there is one other child who does not communicate with her.

She denies any use of illicit drugs, currently or in the past. In theory, by all the available measures, she's considered a low to moderate risk with respect to opioid use. She was started on a few adjuvant analgesic medications as well as a small dose of opioids and recommended to follow-up with a psychologist whom she saw on and off.

Our confirmation test for her UDT came back positive for cocaine. Now, on follow-up conversation with her, she continues to deny illicit drugs. The decision was made to discharge her.

Sometimes it is hard to understand why someone who has been through so much at her age is still using powerful illegal drugs like cocaine or any illicit drugs in light of all the circumstances, while at the same time not ready to receive help. Because of the nature of the case, I decided to place a follow-up phone call to her about a month after we had seen her. She stated on the call that she just got out of a psychiatric unit a few days ago, after being admitted there for about two weeks for attempted suicide. She also stated that she overdosed on the Xanax that was prescribed by her primary care doctor.

The reason she gave for her suicide attempt was that she was overwhelmed by the deaths of her daughter and her son; during this conversation, she stated that his murder was drug-related. In addition, she also admitted to using cocaine. However, she told us that she did that one week prior to her visits to our clinic, and she thought that it would have to be out of her system at the time of her initial visit (I did not question the accuracy of her statement). I, however, asked her about the follow-up appointments she received from the hospital for her psychiatric care. She stated that she was unable to make an appointment with the referrals that were given to her because none of those facilities accepts her healthcare insurance. She was scheduled to see her primary care physician again in two days. So, what should the good doctor do…?

Many of you will agree that there are many issues, questions, and challenges facing this patient. This is in part the reason that cases like these and so many others will depend on not only one physician or provider, but a truly comprehensive multidisciplinary approach even to come close to making a meaningful difference. Stories like this really can drain your energy and motivation, and the desire to continue to help, unless we focus on the greater good that can be accomplished.

However, sometimes there are uplifting moments. It was only a short time ago when **a 58-year-old male** who had back surgery many years ago became a chronic pain patient.

He has had interventional procedures in the past and is currently on opioids. We recently performed epidural steroid injection on him. On his second follow-up visit seen by us, he said: Doc, for the first time in 32 years, I have been without pain for about two weeks.

I didn't know what to do with myself." The joy he felt and the benefit that he got were priceless, and that is what in part helps keep us going. This is not a typical story, and neither is Mary Jane's.

The challenges of the opioid epidemic are real, as are the people. What we face as caring people is how best we can help those who need it and how best to put them on a path where their chances of surviving the opioid epidemic will be much better than before.

This book is a labor of love, and I cherish the opportunity to communicate this information to you. I sincerely hope it will enable you to be of help to your loved ones, to others or even to yourself who may be struggling to find solutions to this powerful opioid epidemic.

I am eternally grateful!

References, Recommended Readings and Resources

1. Definitions.net. https://www.definitions.net/definition/willful%20ignorance. Last visited July 5, 2018.
2. Marc Siegel, M.D.: Fox News. The opioid crisis has a solution --Here it is. July 7, 2018. http://www.foxnews.com/opinion/2018/07/07/dr-marc-siegel-opioid-crisis-has-solution-here-it-is.html. Accessed July 7, 2018.
3. NIH. National Institute of Drug Abuse. Overdose Death Rates Revised August 2018. https://www.drugabuse.gov/related-topics/trends- statistics/ overdose-death-rates. Accessed August 16, 2018.
4. Bill Whitaker. Who's responsible for the opioid epidemic? Doctors or pharmaceutical companies? September 30, 2018. https://www.cbsnews. com/news/jailed-doctor-barry-schultz-interview-opioid-epidemic-60- minutes/. Accessed October 1, 201

Useful Resources and Websites

The **U.S. Department of Health and Human Services (HHS)** functions to enhance and protect the health and well-being of all Americans. It is the government's principal agency for protecting the health and well-being of all Americans.

- https://www.hhs.gov/
- HHS.gov: About the Opioid Epidemic
- https://www.hhs.gov/opioids/about-the-epidemic/

The **Centers for Medicare and Medicaid (CMS)** is responsible for overseeing most of the regulations that are related directly to the healthcare system. It is a federal agency within the Department of Health and Human Services.

- https://www.cms.gov/

The **Centers for Disease Control and Prevention (CDC)** works 24/7 to protect Americans from health and safety threats, both foreign and domestic.

- 800-CDC-INFO (800-232-4636) TTY: 888-232-6348
- Email CDC-INFO
- https://www.cdc.gov

The **Substance Abuse and Mental Health Services Administration (SAMHSA)**'s mission is to reduce the impact of substance abuse and mental illness on America's communities. Congress established the Substance Abuse and Mental Health Services Administration (**SAMHSA**) in 1992 to make substance use and mental disorder information, services, and research more accessible. https://www.samhsa.gov/

- SAMHSA's Behavioral Health Treatment Services Locator
- SAMHSA website (www.dpt.samhsa.gov)

The National Institutes of Health (NIH), a part of the U.S. Department of Health and Human Services, is the nation's medical research agency — making important discoveries that improve health and save lives.

- https://www.nih.gov/about-nih/who-we-are

The National Institute on Drug Abuse (NIDA), is an institute of NIH. NIDA's mission is to advance science on the causes and consequences of drug use and addiction and to apply that knowledge to improve individual and public health.

- https://www.drugabuse.gov/

The Food and Drug Administration (FDA) is responsible for protecting the public health by ensuring the safety, efficacy, and security of human and veterinary drugs, biological products, and medical devices; and by ensuring the safety of our nation's food supply, cosmetics, and products that emit radiation.

- https://www.fda.gov/aboutfda/whatwedo/default.htm

The Drug Enforcement Administration (DEA): controlled substance laws and regulations aim to reduce the supply of and demand for such substances.

- https://www.usa.gov/federal-agencies/drug-enforcement-administration

The Agency for Healthcare Research and Quality (AHRQ)'s mission is to produce evidence to make healthcare safer, higher quality, more accessible, equitable, and affordable, and to work within the U.S. Department of Health and Human Services and with other partners to make sure that the evidence is understood and used.

- https://www.ahrq.gov/cpi/about/mission/index.html

The Joint Commission accredits and certifies healthcare organizations and programs in the United States that have met the standard of care as set by the commission.

- https://www.jointcommission.org/certification/certification_main.aspx

The National Committee for Quality Assurance (NCQA) "exists to improve the quality of health care. We work for better healthcare, better choices and better health".

- https://www.ncqa.org/

The Office of National Drug Control Policy (ONDCP) works to reduce drug use and its consequences by leading and coordinating the development, implementation, and assessment of US drug policy. In addition to its vital ongoing work, ONDCP also provides administrative and financial support to the President's Commission on Combating Drug Addiction and the Opioid Crisis.

- https://www.whitehouse.gov/ondcp/

The Environmental Protection Agency (EPA)'s mission is to protect human health and the environment.

- https://www.epa.gov/aboutepa/our-mission-and-what-we-do

Psychiatry

American Academy of Addiction Psychiatry website (https://www.aaap.org/) The National Alliance on Mental Illness (NAMI) (https://www.nami.org) 3803 N. Fairfax Drive, Suite 100 Arlington, VA 22203

     Main: 703-524-7600

     Member Services: 888-999-6264

     Help Line: 800-950-6264

To report SUSPECTED ADVERSE EVENTS, contact:

The manufacturer of the product taken or FDA MedWatch program by phone at 1-800-FDA-1088 or online at:

- http://www.fda.gov/medwatch/report.htm

Treatment

For information on buprenorphine treatment, contact the SAMHSA Center for Substance Abuse Treatment (CSAT) at 866-BUP-CSAT (866-287-2728) or infobuprenorphine@samhsa.hhs.gov (link sends e-mail).

For information about other medication-assisted treatment (MAT) or the certification of opioid treatment programs (OTPs), contact the SAMHSA Division of Pharmacologic Therapies at 240-276-2700 or otp- extranet@opioid.samhsa.gov (link sends e-mail).

Contact SAMHSA's regional OTP Compliance Officers to determine if an OTP is qualified to provide treatment for substance use disorder.

The American Society of Addiction Medicine:

- https://www.asam.org/ For more information about drug addiction treatment, visit:

- www.drugabuse.gov/publications/principles-drug-addiction-treatment-research- based-guide- third-edition/acknowledgments

For information about drug addiction treatment in the criminal justice system, visit: www.drugabuse.gov/publications/principles-drug-abuse-treatment-criminal-justice-populations/principles

For step-by-step guides for people who think they or a loved one may need treatment, visit: www.drugabuse.gov/related-topics/treatment

Naloxone

For general information about your state's policies regarding naloxone, see the following online resources:

- Naloxone Overdose Prevention Laws Database; Database from the Prescription Drug: http://pdaps.org/datasets/laws-regulating- administration-of-naloxone-1501695139
- Abuse Policy System website: http://pdaps.org/

This database, in the form of an interactive US map from the Prescription Drug Abuse Policy System website, allows users to look up naloxone access laws by state. As of October 2017, the site covers laws passed from 1/1/01 to 7/1/17.

- Legal Interventions to Reduce Overdose Mortality: Naloxone Access and Overdose Good Samaritan Laws.

This fact sheet, from the Network for Public Health Law website, provides a comprehensive table of naloxone access policies by state as of July 15, 2017.

- http://www.ncsl.org/research/civil-and-criminal-justice/drug-overdose-immunity-good-samaritan-laws.aspx

Some Medical and Professional Associations

- Academy of PM& R (AAPM&R) http://www.aapmr.org/
- American College of Sports Medicine
- National Stroke Association
- Neurosurgeon.com
- American Association of Neuromuscular and Electrodiagnostic Medicine
- Academy of Integrative Pain Management https://www.integrativepainmanagement.org/
- Academic Orthopedic Society
- The American Society of Regional Anesthesia and Pain Medicine (ASRA) https://www.asra.com/
- American Academy of Orthopedic Surgeons
- Interventional Orthopedic Foundation https://interventionalorthopedics.org/
- American Academy of Family Medicine
- Spine Intervention Society https://www.spineintervention.org
- American Academy of Pain Medicine
- National American Spine Society
- American Society of Interventional Pain Physicians (ASIPP) http://www.asipp. org/
- American Academy of Pediatrics
- American Academy of Neurological Surgeons
- American Medical Association
- American Society for Surgery
- American Society of Internal Medicine
- Society of General Internal Medicine
- Radiological Society of North America
- American Academy of Neurology
- American Board of Pain Medicine: http://www.abpm.org/
- American Society of Interventional Pain Physicians: http://www.asipp. org/
- American Chiropractic Association: https://www.acatoday.org/
- American Dental Association: https://www.ada.org/
- American Physical Therapy Association: http://www.apta.org/
- American Society of Addiction Medicine: https://www.asam.org/

Other Useful Sites

- Alcoholic Anonymous: https://www.aa.org/
- Harm Reduction Coalition: https://harmreduction.org/
- The National Domestic Hotline: https://www.thehotline.org/
- National Suicide Prevention Lifeline: https://suicidepreventionlifeline. org/
- Help and Resources | Drug Overdose | CDC Injury Center: https://www. cdc.gov/drugoverdose/prevention/help.html
- Narcotics Anonymous: https://www.na.org/

Appendices

A-E

APPENDIX A

How to calculate **Morphine Milligrams Equivalent (MME)** daily dose, also called **Morphine Equivalent Dose (MED)** daily or **Morphine Equivalent Daily (MED)** dose. The calculation of MME uses morphine as the reference opioid base on the strength or potency of other opioids. There are many different types of methods and/or applications that are available for calculations. There are therefore different results that are obtained, sometimes depending on the applications or methods that are used. So be aware of the applications that you can install on your smartphone or tablets, as well as the various computer programs that are available, and make sure that whatever you use reconcile with some known standard.

The CDC has a conversion table which is available for use. Although it does not cover some opioids, it still forms a significant reference point from which to determine the MME of each patient that are prescribed opioids. The table and the conversion factors are shown below.

Calculating Morphine Milligram Equivalents (MME)	
OPIOID (doses in mg/day except where noted)	**CONVERSION FACTOR**
Codeine	0.15
Fentanyl transdermal (in mcg/hr.)	2.4
Hydrocodone	1
Hydromorphone	4
Methadone	
1-20 mg/day	4
21-40 mg/day	8
41-60mg/day	10
$\geq 61 - 80$ mg/day	12
Morphine	1
Oxycodone	1.5
Oxymorphone	3

These dose conversions are estimated and cannot account for all individual differences in genetics and pharmacokinetics (CDC protocol).

1. **Determine** the total daily amount of each opioid the patient takes.
2. **Convert** each to MMEs—multiply the dose for each opioid by the conversion factor.
3. **Add** them together.

Methadone and Fentanyl seem to vary in the results calculated in a number of different programs.

Buprenorphine, a partial agonist, is not included in the CDC calculations, but most calculations are done with a conversion factor of **1.8** (for each daily microgram unit).

Tramadol has a conversion factor of **0.10**.

Reference

Centers for Disease Control and Prevention. https://www.cdc.gov/drugoverdose/pdf/calculating_total_daily_dose-a.pdf. Accessed May 30, 2018.

APPENDIX B

DEA DRUGS (CONTROLLED SUBSTANCES) CLASSIFICATION

This section included a table showing how drugs are generally classified by the Drug Enforcement Administration (**DEA**).

CLASS	CRITERIA	EXAMPLES OF DRUGS
Schedule I	No currently accepted medical use and a high potential for abuse.	Some examples of Schedule I drugs are: heroin, lysergic acid diethylamide (LSD), marijuana (cannabis), 3,4-methylenedioxymethamphetamine (ecstasy), methaqualone, and peyote
Schedule II	High potential for abuse, with use potentially leading to severe psychological or physical dependence. These drugs are also considered dangerous	Combination products with less than 15 milligrams of hydrocodone per dosage unit (Vicodin), cocaine, methamphetamine, methadone, hydromorphone (Dilaudid), meperidine (Demerol), oxycodone (OxyContin), fentanyl, Dexedrine, Adderall, and Ritalin
Schedule III	Moderate to low potential for physical and psychological dependence. Schedule III drugs abuse potential is less than Schedule I and Schedule II drugs but more than Schedule IV	Products containing less than 90 milligrams of codeine per dosage unit (Tylenol with codeine), ketamine, anabolic steroids, testosterone
Schedule IV	Low potential for abuse and low risk of dependence	Xanax, Soma, Darvon, Darvocet, Valium, Ativan, Talwin, Ambien, Tramadol

Schedule V	Lower potential for abuse than Schedule IV and consists of preparations containing limited quantities of certain narcotics. Schedule V drugs are generally used for antidiarrheal, antitussive, and analgesic purposes.	Cough preparations with less than 200 milligrams of codeine or per 100 milliliters (Robitussin AC), Lomotil, Motofen, Lyrica, Parepectolin

This also is very useful in your understanding of the potential danger and usefulness of some of these substances/drugs.

DEA Schedule I-V classification of narcotics and controlled drugs.

The Controlled Substance Act of 1970 in part empowered the DEA to classify drugs/control substances. The drugs/substances are classified as indicated in the table above into five classes or schedules depending upon the substance/drug's acceptable medical use and their potential for abuse or to cause dependence. Drugs or substances can be added, or class/schedule changed depending on the current or new information.

APPENDIX C

CDC 2016 Summary Guideline for Chronic Pain

GUIDELINE FOR PRESCRIBING OPIOIDS FOR CHRONIC PAIN
IMPROVING PRACTICE THROUGH RECOMMENDATIONS

CDC's Guideline for Prescribing Opioids for Chronic Pain is intended to improve communication between providers and patients about the risks and benefits of opioid therapy for chronic pain, improve the safety and effectiveness of pain treatment, and reduce the risks associated with long-term opioid therapy, including opioid use disorder and overdose. The Guideline is not intended for patients who are inactive cancer treatment, palliative care, or end-of-life care.

DETERMINING WHEN TO INITIATE OR CONTINUE
OPIOIDS FOR CHRONIC PAIN

- Nonpharmacologic therapy and nonopioid pharmacologic therapy are preferred for chronic pain. Clinicians should consider opioid therapy only if expected benefits for both pain and function are anticipated to outweigh risks to the patient. If opioids are used, they should be combined with nonpharmacologic therapy and nonopioid pharmacologic therapy, as appropriate.
- Before starting opioid therapy for chronic pain, clinicians should establish treatment goals with all patients, including realistic goals for pain and function, and should consider how opioid therapy will be discontinued if benefits do not outweigh risks. Clinicians should continue opioid therapy only if there is clinically meaningful improvement in pain and function that outweighs risks to patient safety.
- Before starting and periodically during opioid therapy, clinicians should discuss with patients known risks and realistic benefits of opioid therapy and patient and clinician responsibilities for managing therapy.

CLINICAL REMINDERS

- Opioids are not first-line or routine therapy for chronic pain
- Establish and measure goals for pain and function
- Discuss benefits and risks and availability of non-opioid therapies with patient.

OPIOID SELECTION, DOSAGE, DURATION, FOLLOW- UP, AND DISCONTINUATION

- When starting opioid therapy for chronic pain, clinicians should prescribe immediate-release opioids instead of extended-release/long- acting (ER/LA) opioids.

- When opioids are started, clinicians should prescribe the lowest effective dosage. Clinicians should use caution when prescribing opioids at any dosage, should carefully reassess evidence of individual benefits and risks when considering increasing dosage to ≥50 morphine milligram equivalents (MME)/day, and should avoid increasing dosage to ≥90 MME/day or carefully justify a decision to titrate dosage to ≥90 MME/ day.

- Long-term opioid use often begins with treatment of acute pain. When opioids are used for acute pain, clinicians should prescribe the lowest effective dose of immediate-release opioids and should prescribe no greater quantity than needed for the expected duration of pain severe enough to require opioids. Three days or less will often be sufficient; more than seven days will rarely be needed. Clinicians should evaluate benefits and harms with patients within 1 to 4 weeks of starting opioid therapy for chronic pain or of dose escalation.

- Clinicians should evaluate benefits and harms of continued therapy with patients every 3 months or more frequently. If benefits do not outweigh harms of continued opioid therapy, clinicians should optimize other therapies and work with patients to taper opioids to lower dosages or to taper and discontinue opioids.

CLINICAL REMINDERS

- Use immediate-release opioids when starting
- Start low and go slow
- When opioids are needed for acute pain, prescribe no more than needed
- Do not prescribe ER/LA opioids for acute pain
- Follow-up and re-evaluate risk of harm; reduce dose or taper and discontinue if needed.

ASSESSING RISK ANDADDRESSING HARMS OF OPIOID USE

- Before starting and periodically during continuation of opioid therapy, clinicians should evaluate risk factors for opioid-related harms. Clinicians should incorporate into the management plan strategies to mitigate risk, including considering offering naloxone when factors that increase risk for opioid overdose, such as history of overdose, history of substance use disorder, higher opioid dosages (≥50 MME/day), or concurrent benzodiazepine use, are present.
- Clinicians should review the patient's history of controlled substance prescriptions using state prescription drug monitoring program (PDMP) data to determine whether the patient is receiving opioid dosages or dangerous combinations that put him or her at high risk for overdose. Clinicians should review PDMP data when starting opioid therapy for chronic pain and periodically during opioid therapy for chronic pain, ranging from every prescription to every 3 months.
- When prescribing opioids for chronic pain, clinicians should use urine drug testing before starting opioid therapy and consider urine drug testing at least annually to assess for prescribed medications as well as other controlled prescription drugs and illicit drugs.
- Clinicians should avoid prescribing opioid pain medication and benzodiazepines concurrently whenever possible.
- Clinicians should offer or arrange evidence-based treatment (usually medication-assisted treatment with buprenorphine or methadone in combination with behavioral therapies) for patients with opioid use disorder.

CLINICAL REMINDERS

- Evaluate risk factors for opioid-related harms
- Check PDMP for high dosages and prescriptions from other providers
- Use urine drug testing to identify prescribed substances and undisclosed use
- Avoid concurrent benzodiazepine and opioid prescribing
- Arrange treatment for opioid use disorder if needed

LEARN MORE | www.cdc.gov/drugoverdose/prescribing/guideline.html

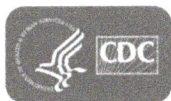

U.S. Department of
Health and Human Services
Centers for Disease
Control and Prevention

APPENDIX D

Table of Different Drug Classes, Street Names, Generic Names, Route of Ingestion, Appearance, and Schedule

Tables of different drug classes, ranging from opioids, central nervous system depressants, central nervous system stimulants, hallucinogens, psychoactive drugs and substances that are commonly abuse or have the potential for abuse or misuse.

This is intended for use primarily as a reference, and will also be helpful to you in understanding and appreciating the different types of drugs/substances that are available. This is of course only a partial list of the numerous compounds that are available. So, familiarize yourself with them and some of the different street names that are associated with these drugs.

PRESCRIPTION OPIOIDS

NARCOTICS	TRADE NAMES	STREET NAMES	APPEARANCES	ROUTE OF INGESTION	SCHEDULE
Buprenorphine	Suboxone, Buprenex, and Subutex,	Bupe	Tablets	Swallowed, skin patch, injected	III
Codeine	Codeine (various brand names)	Captain Cody, Cody, Lean, Schoolboy, Sizzurp, Purple Drank.	Tablet, capsule, liquid	Injected, swallowed (often mixed with soda and flavorings)	IV
Fentanyl	Duragesic, Actiq, Fentora, Sublimaze	China White, Dance Fever Lollipop, Perc-O-Pop, China White, Mexican Brown Apache, China Girl, Friend, Goodfella, Jackpot, Murder 8, Tango and Cash, TNT	Crushed, cake-like, crumbly, powdered, patch tablets, film, buccal tablets	Swallowed, injected, skin patch snorted	II
Heroine (Not prescribed in the US)	No commercial name	Brown sugar, China White, Dope, H, Horse, Junk, Skag, Skink, Smack, White Horse	White or brownish powder or black sticky substance is known as "black tar heroin	Smoked, snorted, injected	I
Hydrocodone	Vicodin, Vicoprofen, Reprexain, Ibudone	Vikes, Codone, Hydro, Viko, Norco, Watson-387	Tablets, capsules, liquid	Swallowed snorted, injected	II
Hydromorphone	Dilaudid	Footballs, Juice, Dillies, smak	Liquid, suppository, tablets	Ingested, rectal, swallowed, snorted	II
Meperidine	Demerol	Demmies, Pain Killer	White crystalline substance, liquid, tablets	Snorted, Oral, injected	II
Methadone	Dolophine, Methadose	Dollie, Amidone, Fizzies, With MDMA: Chocolate Chip Cookies	Tablets, solution	Swallowed, snorted, injected	II

Morphine (M), Morphine Sulfate	MS Contin, Duramorph,	M, Miss Emma, Atom Bomb, Monkey, White Stuff	White powder or crystals, clear liquid, tablets, capsules, suppository	Swallowed, nasal, smoked, injected	II
Oxycodone	Roxicodone, Roxicef, OxyContin, Percodan, Percocet	O, C., Roxi, Molly, Perk, Oxycet, Oxycotton, Oxy, Hillbilly Heroin, Percs	White to off-white powder, as tablets, liquid, capsule	Swallowed Chewed, snorted, injected	II
Oxymorphone	Opana Numorphan,	Biscuits, Blue Heaven, Blues, Mrs. O, O Bomb, Octagons, Stop Signs	Tablets	Swallowed, snorted, injected	
Tapentadol	Nucynta, Tapal, Palexia	Cha Cha	Oral suspension, tablets	Swallowed, snorted, injected	II
Tramadol	Ultram®, Ultracet, ConZip, Ryzolt, Rybix ODT and	Chill Pills, Ultras	Tablets, capsules	Swallowed, snorted injected	III

CENTRAL NERVOUS SYSTEM DEPRESSANTS					
GENERIC NAMES	TRADE NAMES	STREET NAMES	APPEARANCES	ROUTE OF INGESTION	SCHEDULE
BARBITURATES:					
Amobarbital	Amytal, Stadadorm	Barbs, Blues, Blue Dolls, Rainbows, Nebbies, Downers, Reds, Red Devils, Phennies, Red Birds, Reds, Tooies, Yellow Jackets, Yellows	Capsule, powder, tablets, solution	Swallowed snorted, injected	II, III, IV
Butabarbital	Butisol				
Butalbital	Fiorinal				
Pentobarbital	Luminal, Neodorm				
Phenobarbital	Nembutal				
Secobarbital	Seconal				
BENZODIAZEPINE:					
Alprazolam	Xanax	Candy, Benzo, Bzd, Nerve Pills, Goofballs, Valley Girl, Heavenly Blues, Stupefy , Downers, Sleeping Pills, Tranks	Capsule, powder, tablets, solution	Swallowed snorted, injected	IV
Chlordiazepoxide	Librium				
Clonazepam	Klonopin				
Clorazepate	Tranxene				
Diazepam	Valium				
Flurazepam	Dalmane				
Lorazepam	Ativan, Tavor, Tamestra				
Oxazepam	Serax				
Temazepam	Restoril				
Triazolam	Halcion				
ROHYPNOL (Flunitrazepam)	Flunitrazepam, Rohypnol®	Circles, Date Rape Drug, Forget Pill, Forget-Me Pill, La Rocha, Lunch Money, Mexican Valium, Mind Eraser, Pingus, R2, Reynolds, Rib, Roach, Roach 2, Roaches, Roachies, Roapies, Rochas Dos, Roofies, Rope, Rophies, Row-shay, Ruffies, Trip-and-Fall, Wolfies	Tablet	Swallowed (as a pill or as dissolved in a drink), snorted, injected	IV

CENTRAL NERVOUS SYSTEM STIMULANTS					
GENERIC NAMES	TRADE NAMES	STREET NAMES	APPEARANCES	ROUTE OF INGESTION	SCHEDULE
Amphetamine	Adderall, Benzedrine, Dexedrine	Bennies, Black Beauties, Crosses, Hearts, LA Turnaround, Speed, Truck Drivers, Uppers	Tablets, capsules, solution	Oral, nasal, smoked, injected	II
Bath Salts	Cathinone, Methylenedioxypyro valerone, Mephedrone	Flakka, Ivory Wave, Plant Fertilizer, Vanilla Sky, Energy-1, Red Dove, White Dove, Blue Silk, Zoom, Hurricane, Aura, Alpha PVC	White, tan, or brown colored powdery substance	Ingested, snorted, smoked, or injected	I
Cocaine	None	Blow, Rock Bump, Coke, Snow, Crack, Flake, Toot, Cola, White Girl	White Powder, whitish rock crystal	Oral, nasal smoked, injected	II
Ecstasy/MDMA	None	Peace, Uppers, Lovers Speed, Ecstasy, X-Tc, Adam, Skittles, Tabs, Molly	Colorful tabs, liquid, white powder, capsules, tablets	Oral, injected, snorted.	I
Methamphetamine	Desoxyn, Methedrine	Crank, Glass Doe, Crystal, Speed, Ice, Meth, Tina	Tablets, capsules, solution, crystal meth glass, white powder	Oral, smoked, nasal, injected	II
Methylphenidate	Ritalin, Concerta	JIF, MPH, Skippy, The Smart Drug, Vitamin R, Diet Coke, Kiddy Coke, R Pop, Study, Pineapple, Poor Man's Cocaine,	Tablets, capsules, patches, and liquid	Snorted, smoked, Oral (dissolve in beverage) Chewed, injected	II

HALLUCINOGENS					
GENERIC NAMES	**TRADE NAMES**	**STREET NAMES**	**APPEARANCES**	**ROUTE OF INGESTION**	**SCHEDULE**
Alcohol	Wine, Beer, Liquor	Booze, Brew	Color or colorless liquid	Oral	N
Dextromethorphan	Many: Vicks 44, Creomulsion, Delsym, Tussin Pediatric, DM	Robotripping, Robo, Skittles, Triple C, DXM, Syrup,	Syrup, Tablets	Oral, syrup injection	N
Ketamine	Ketalar	Super K, Kit-Kat, Kitty, Special K, Vitamin K, Cat Valium	White powder, clear or cream-colored liquid	Injected, mixed in beverage, sniffed, snorted, smoked (powder added to tobacco or marijuana cigarettes), swallowed	III
Lysergic Acid Diethylamide (LSD)	Delysid	Acid, Dots, Window Panes, Blotter, Blue Heaven, Cubes, Microdot, Yellow Sunshine, Sugar Cubes	White, odorless powder, tablets, capsules, solids, liquids, sugar cubes, gelatin, blotting paper	Oral	I
Mescaline (Peyote)	None	Mesc, Cactus, Buttons	Natural-looking fresh or dried "buttons", tablets or capsules	Oral, Chewed, nasal, smoked, injected	I
Phencyclidine (PCP)	Sernyl, Sernylan	Angel Dust, boat Space Cadet, Pcp, Hog Dust, White Devil, peace pill	White or colored powder, tablets or capsules, colorless crystals, clear liquid	Oral, nasal, smoked, swallowed, injected. Added to marijuana, mint	I

CANNABINOIDS

GENERIC NAMES	TRADE NAMES	STREET NAMES	APPEARANCES	ROUTE OF INGESTION	SCHEDULE
Cannabis, Marijuana, Hashish	Marinol, Dronabinol	Blunt, Bud, Dope, Ganja, Grass, Green, Herb, Joint, Mary Jane, Pot, Reefer, Sinsemilla, Skunk, Smoke, Trees, Weed; Hashish: Boom, Gangster, Hash, Hemp	Seeds, oils, leaves, capsules, buds, liquid	Mixed in food or teat, smoked, oral	I
Synthetic Cannabinoids	JWH-018, UR-144, XLR-11 (5-F-UR144), AB-PINACA, 5-F-AB-PINACA, AB-CHMINACA, APP-CHMINACA, AB-FUBINACA, AB-CHMICA, ADBICA, and 5-F-ABICA to name a few	K2, Spice Gold, Spice, Sdiamond, Yucatan Fire, Genie, Fire N Ice, Black Mamba, Bombay Blue, Zombie World, The Moon, Bliss	Powder, plant extracts	Snorted, smoked, sold as incense, potpourri	I

MUSCLE RELAXANT

GENERIC NAMES	TRADE NAMES	STREET NAMES	APPEARANCES	ROUTE OF INGESTION	SCHEDULE
Carisoprodol	Soma, Prosoma	Ds, Dance, Las Vegas Cocktail	Pills	Bumped, injected, smoked	IV

OVER THE COUNTER DRUGS

GENERIC NAMES	TRADE NAMES	STREET NAMES	APPEARANCES	ROUTE OF INGESTION	SCHEDULE
Dextromethorphan	Many: Vicks 44, Creomulsion, Delsym, Tussin Pediatric, DM	Robotripping, Robo, Skittles, Triple C, DXM, Syrup,	Syrup, Tablets	Oral, syrup injection	N
Kratom	No commercial name	Herbal Speedball, Biak-biak, Ketum, Kahuam, Ithang, Thom.	Fresh or dried leaves, powder, liquid, gum	Chewed (whole leaves), eaten (mixed in food or brewed as tea), occasionally smoked	N
Loperamide	Imodium	None	Tablet, capsule, liquid	Swallowed	N
Inhalants	Various	Poppers, Snappers, Whippets, Laughing gas	Paint thinners or removers, degreasers, dry cleaning fluids, gasoline, lighter fluids, correction fluids, permanent markers, electronic cleaners and freeze sprays, glue, spray paint, hair or deodorant sprays, fabric protector sprays, aerosol computer cleaning products, vegetable oil sprays, butane lighter, propane tanks, whipped cream aerosol containers, refrigerant gases, ether, chloroform, halothane, nitrous oxide	Inhaled through the nose and mouth	N

Reference: National Institute on Drug Abuse. Commonly abused drugs charts. https://www.drugabuse.gov/drugs-abuse/commonly-abused-drugs- charts. Accessed April 2, 2018.

APPENDIX E

FOSTER'S OPIOID CLASSIFICATIONADDICTION STATUS (FOCAS)

This section will provide a brief explanation of the **Foster's Opioid Classification Addiction Status** or FOCAS. For those interested in a more extended version of this classification, please refer to the publication (book) called *Foster's Opioid Classification Addiction Status Guide*. This was published in January 2019. Author: D Terrence Foster.

The **FOCAS** is a nomenclature (naming) or grouping of every one of us into a class. This allows for easier characterization of individuals/patients or potential users and users of opioids. This flowchart (algorithms) will enable comparable language and descriptions among providers in the healthcare field. This can also help with treatment stratification or protocols. In general, this has the potential to simplify communications between professionals as well as between professionals and their patients. **Flowchart (algorithm) for FOCAS** is on the next page.

THE FLOWCHART (ALGORITHM) FOR FOCAS GUIDE
FOSTER'S OPIOID ADDICTION CLASSIFICATION STATUS

ACUTE PAIN

CLASS ZERO (Normal)

CHRONIC PAIN

Minor Injury, Auto, Work Comp, Procedure, Surgery, Ortho, Other

Minor Injury, Auto, Work Comp, Procedure, Surgery, Ortho, Other

NN   1A   1C   N/NN

Well

1B   N

Well

Well

NN   2A   2C   N/NN

Well

2B   N

Well

Well

Not Well

Not Well

Well

Not Well

Not Well

Not Well

Well

Not Well

N

N

RX Diversion

5 X A

5 X B

5 X C

RX

RX Supplies

PAIN SPECIALISTS

N

3C   3B   3A

Not Well

Not Well

Well

N

DEALERS

5 D

4C   4B   4A

Not Well

Not Well

Well

Maintained, Not Addicted

SUPPLIERS

5 S

Well, Treated

5A

ADDICTION

Treated   5B   5C   Not Treated

Overdose/Jail/Death

Overdose/Jail/Death

N – Opioid,
NN – No Opioid

REGARDING FOSTER'S OPIOID CLASSIFICATION ADDICTION STATUS (FOCAS)

1. **Class 0, 1 and 2** are opioid naïve, these are users with no opioid use or limited opioid use such as prior prescriptions for minor procedures that resulted in small quantities of opioids prescribed (example: from dentists, podiatrists, etc.)

2. **Class 3** has a history of opioid use, with initial intervention by consultants, they are not addicted to opioids, some may have developed tolerance.

3. **Class 4** has extended opioids use with or without specialists, some of them may have opioid tolerance or dependence.

4. **Class 5** this class has the **Addiction Groups 5A, 5B and 5C** (Addicts or Opioid Use Disorder groups), the **Illegal Groups 5XA, 5XB and 5XC**, as well as the **Dealers Groups 5XD (A, B, and C),** and **Suppliers Groups 5XS (A, B, and C).**

5. The group designated as "C" has a history of psychiatric, psychological, behavioral disorder, cognitive impairment or non-opioids substance abuse history in Groups One and Two. However, Classes 3 and 4 are combinations of the preceding Classes. Therefore, Groups 3A and 4A, (well groups) now have patients previously designated as "C" in Groups One and Two (patients with psychiatric disorders/substance abuse, etc. do get well and can be stable on or off opioids also). Groups 3B, 4B, 5A and 5B are the treated groups without psychiatric, cognitive or non-opioid substance abuse disorders.

6. Treatments referred to range from limited therapy and or medications to multidisciplinary approach intervention and or medications.

7. There are multiple overlaps and when in doubt patients should be placed at the higher level (more complex) with respect to treatment and classification.

8. Most of the addictions, overdoses and opioid deaths that occur in the United States are likely to come from the Groups 5XA, 5XB, and 5XC. These are primarily the none prescription opioids (diverted legally prescribed opioids) and illegal opioids such as heroin and illicitly manufactured fentanyl. It may sometimes be difficult to establish wellness accurately with respect to 5XA and 5XB and 5XC in general.

9. If the drugs dealers and suppliers become users of illegal opioids and or illegal non-opioid drugs their classification will be 5XD (A, B or C) and 5XS (A, B or C) respectively. The associated table referred to as the **FOCAS TABLE** on the next page also explains the flowchart.

FOCAS TABLE

Time	Class	Groups		
None	**ZERO**	-	Normal	-
Less than three mo., acute opioid naïve	**ONE**	**1A:** treatment without opioids, well	**1B:** treatment with opioids	**1C:** treatment with or without opioids, psychiatry, etc.
3 mo. -1yr plus, chronic opioid naïve	**TWO**	**2A:** treatment without opioids, well	**2B:** treatment with opioids	**2C:** treatment with or without an opioid, psych., etc.
1-2 yrs., chronic, opioids	**THREE**	**3A:** treatment with opioids, well	**3B:** treatment with opioids, not well	**3C:** treatment, well, not well, psych, etc.
>2yrs, chronic, opioids	**FOUR**	**4A:** treatment with opioids, well	**4B:** treatment with opioids, not well	**4C:** treatment, not well, psych, etc.
>2yrs, chronic, opioids	**FIVE (Addiction groups, use illicit opioids/Rx)**	**5A:** well, not well. Usually have good support, money/social network	**5B:** well, not well, OD, jail. Have some level of support.	**5C:** not well, Psych, etc. No treatment, OD, jail, death? Have poor support structure.
Undefined	**FIVE (Illicit Groups)**	**These are the groups with multiple unknown factors** Without medical doctors/services or sense of direction Extremely difficult to treat, numerous unknown factors. Very risky.		
	X	**5XA**	Has no pain, using illegal prescription drugs	
	X	**5XB**	Has pain, using illegal prescription drugs	
	X	**5XC**	Has pain or no pain, using illegal prescription & illegal none-prescription drug, psychiatry, etc.	
	X	**5XD (A, B or C)**	Illegal Drug dealers	
	X	**5XS (A, B or C)**	Illegal Drug suppliers	

Index

BRIEF SUMMARY OF THE OPIOID EPIDEMIC CONSUMERS & HEALTHCARE GUIDE

This book looks at how the opioid epidemic started and where we are now. We examined and explained the causes of the opioid epidemic and who are most likely responsible, as we look at prescription drugs and the doctors and providers who write these prescriptions. The impact of legal and illegal opioids and their contribution to the opioid epidemic are discussed. Also, non-opioid drugs, which are also a major contributing factor to the opioid epidemic, are considered.

The significance of diversions of opioids and controlled substances are presented. The impact of the opioid epidemic on family and loved ones, including teens and young adults, is also presented, as well as some of the obstacles to available treatment.

Appropriate medical, nonmedical intervention, and treatment as well as the obstacles faced by those of us who work with chronic and acute pain patients are elaborated on at length with an emphasis on addiction treatment and prevention. Alternative therapies such as marijuana, non-traditional treatments, and some controversial programs are also examined. The importance of naloxone is thoroughly covered. As we move forward, we looked at what can be done, and some of the things that are being done in other countries that are helpful in their fight against the opioid crisis. We also looked at what is being done in our country by various sectors, including but not limited to the government, providers, and healthcare insurance companies.

The importance of opioid use in our society is discussed, along with the need for continuing opioid treatment despite the number of deaths it has caused.

This book provides a relatively simple approach to a very complex problem; as well as information that will create a better understanding by consumers, the public as a whole, and healthcare providers/physicians of some of the challenges involved with opioid use, treatment and addiction. This book is intended for consumers and the general public, as well as healthcare providers. Particularly those mainly engaged in primary care and service treatment of patients who are potential users of opioids, and those who are already on opioids and other controlled substances.

Author: Dr. D. Terrence Foster

ABOUT THE AUTHOR
D. Terrence Foster, M.D., MA, FAAPMR, DABPM

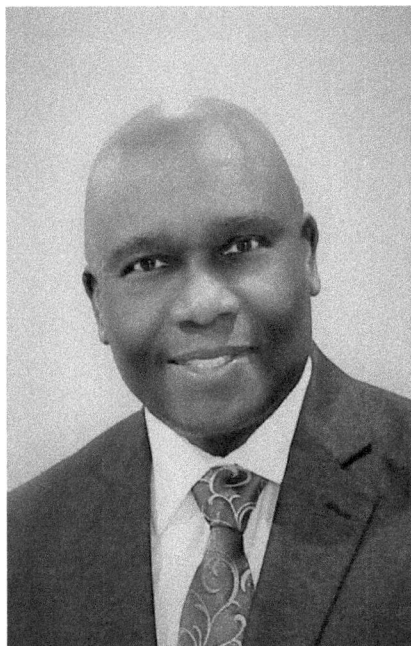

Dr. Foster graduated from The Albert Einstein College of Medicine of Yeshiva University, New York, where he earned his Doctor of Medicine. At the City University of New York, he received a Master's Degree in Chemistry and from the University of the West Indies, a Bachelor of Science - BS (Hons) in Chemistry. His medical training was completed at Jacobi Medical Center/Albert Einstein Hospital, New York - Internship. Residency at New York University Medical Center/ Rusk Institute of Rehabilitation Medicine- Physical Medicine & Rehabilitation and Medical College of Wisconsin, Milwaukee: Fellowship, Electrodiagnostic Medicine (EMG).

Dr. Foster worked as an Attending Physician and Clinical Instructor at Emory University Hospitals, Wesley Woods Geriatric Hospital and Center for Rehab Medicine. He is a former Medical Director for The Rehabilitation Center at Southern Regional Health System, Riverdale, GA, where he served for ten years.

Dr. Foster has medical staff privileges at several medical centers in the state of Georgia. He is currently the Medical Director for the Center for Pain and Rehab Medicine in Stockbridge, GA, where his primary focus is Interventional Pain and Addiction Medicine.

He is Board Certified in Physical Medicine and Rehabilitation, and a fellow of the American Academy of Physical Medicine and Rehabilitation. He is also a Diplomate of the American Board of Physical Medicine and Rehabilitation. He is Board Certified in Pain Medicine and a Diplomate of the American Board of Pain Medicine.

Dr. Foster is the author or co-author of several scientific articles and the author of the book *Foster's Opioid Addiction Classification Status Guide*. He also previously hosted a radio show called "The Doctor Show." He is a member of several medical associations.

Visit his website at: DTERRENCEFOSTER.COM

Photo by: Atlanta Photographers Network.

FOSTER'S OPIOID CLASSIFICATION ADDICTION STATUS (FOCAS) GUIDE

DETERMINING OPIOID USERS STATUS AND TREATMENT OPTIONS

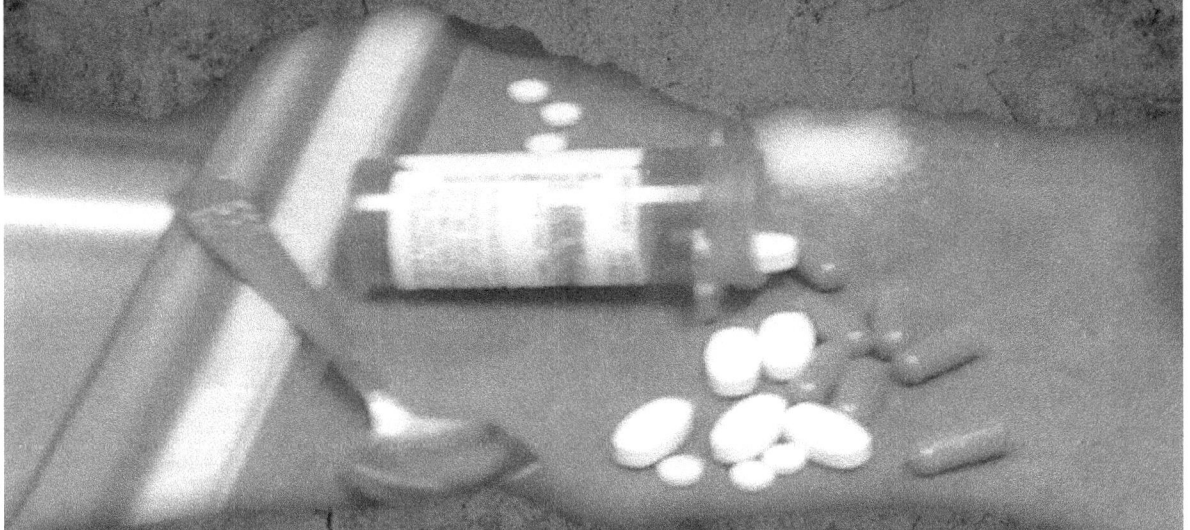

D. TERRENCE FOSTER, M.D., FAAPMR, DABPM

GLOBAL HEALTH AND CONSORTIUM PUBLISHING

GHC

www.ingramcontent.com/pod-product-compliance
Lightning Source LLC
Chambersburg PA
CBHW081412270326
41931CB00015B/3252